EFFECTIVE
COMMUNICATION
SKILLS FOR HEALTH
PROFESSIONALS

FORTHCOMING TITLES

Occupational Therapy for the Brain-Injured Adult
Jo Clark-Wilson and Gordon Muir Giles

Visual Impairment: Perspectives in practice
Jane Hutchinson

Assessment in Occupational Therapy
Greg Kelly

Early Identification of Language Impairment in Children
James Law

Speech and Language Problems in Children
Dilys A. Treharne

THERAPY IN PRACTICE SERIES

Edited by Jo Campling

This series of books is aimed at 'therapists' concerned with rehabilitation in a very broad sense. The intended audience particularly includes occupational therapists, physiotherapists and speech therapists, but many titles will also be of interest to nurses, psychologists, medical staff, social workers, teachers or volunteer workers. Some volumes are interdisciplinary, others are aimed at one particular profession. All titles will be comprehensive but concise, and practical but with due reference to relevant theory and evidence. They are not research monographs but focus on professional practice, and will be of value to both students and qualified personnel.

Effective Communication Skills for Health Professionals

Philip Burnard

Director of Postgraduate Nursing Studies, University of Wales College of Medicine, Cardiff, Wales and Honorary Lecturer, Institute for Higher Professional Education for Health Care Professions, Hogeschool Midden Nederland, Utrecht, The Netherlands

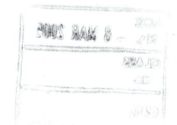

CHAPMAN & HALL
London · New York · Tokyo · Melbourne · Madras

Published by Chapman & Hall, 2–6 Boundary Row, London SE1 8HN

Chapman & Hall, 2–6 Boundary Row, London SE1 8HN, UK

Chapman & Hall, 29 West 35th Street, New York NY10001, USA

Chapman & Hall Japan, Thomson Publishing Japan, Hirakawacho Nemoto Building, 7F, 1-7-11 Hirakawa-cho, Chiyoda-ku, Tokyo 102, Japan

Chapman & Hall Australia, Thomas Nelson Australia, 102 Dodds Street, South Melbourne, Victoria 3205, Australia

Chapman & Hall India, R. Seshadri, 32 Second Main Road, CTT East, Madras 600 035, India

First edition 1992

© 1992 Philip Burnard

Typeset in 10/12pt Times by Excel Typesetters Company, Hong Kong
Printed in Great Britain by St Edmundsbury Press, Bury St. Edmunds, Suffolk.

ISBN 0 412 40870 8

A catalogue record for this book is available from the British Library

Library of Congress Cataloging-in-Publication data available

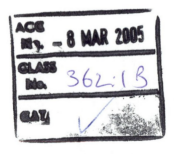

Contents

Introduction

We are all communicating, nearly all of the time. What we say, how we say it, what we wear, how we sit and so on: all of these things are aspects of how we present ourselves to other people. We may not be able to do anything about that. What we can improve, is our *means* of communication. We can do much to improve the way we communicate. Consider the following situations:

- You are working with a colleague who is senior to you and whom you don't like very much;
- You are interviewing a teenage boy about his family;
- You are 'off duty' and having a drink with some of your colleagues;
- You are presenting a short paper to a conference on some research that you have just completed;
- You are asked to write a report on what you see as health care priorities in your area;
- You are at home with the person you live with or with your family and a client rings to talk to you.

In each case you are communicating. But do you communicate easily and effectively in each of these situations? Which situation would be easiest for you and which would you try to avoid? Would you be 'yourself' in each situation or would you have to bluff a little in some of them? This book is about some of the skills involved in coping with these and other health care situations.

Effective Communication Skills for Health Professionals is about practical ways of enhancing communication between health professionals and their patients or clients and between those professionals and their colleagues. Its aim is to encourage you to think about how you present yourself to others in everyday life. There is no right way, no single method of ensuring that you will be understood by others. There are a lot of straightforward methods of helping you to communicate more effectively. This book highlights some of those ways and points to some obstacles that may get in your way.

WHO THIS BOOK IS FOR

Communication is a vital aspect of health care. Just look around you at your colleagues and notice the degree to which they communicate effectively. More painfully, perhaps, look at yourself as you talk to patients, clients or colleagues. Most of us can benefit from a little self-analysis and a bit of rethinking about taken-for-granted aspects of how we come across to others.

This book is for all students in the health care professions and at all levels: in basic training or education, at diploma, graduate and post-graduate levels. It will be of use to doctors, nurses, occupational therapists, speech therapists, social workers and voluntary workers — anyone who is intimately involved in managing, caring for or working with others.

WHAT IS IN THE BOOK

The book focuses on clusters of skills. Those communication skills are identified under the following headings:

- educational skills
- therapeutic skills
- organizational skills
- personal skills

Part One opens with a chapter which discusses teaching skills and will be useful to anyone who has to teach colleagues or clients in any setting. Whilst there are a variety of philosophies of teaching and learning, many of the basic structural aspects of teaching can be identified easily. The approach taken in this chapter is concerned with adult teaching and learning.

In the second chapter, presentational skills are addressed. Many health professionals find that it is only a matter of time before they are called upon to talk to a fairly large audience — at a conference or presentation. This chapter explores ways of making such presentations effective. The skills involved here will also be helpful when you have to present cases or plans to colleagues or managers in various settings.

The first part of the book closes with a chapter on computers and computing skills: what to look for and what computers can do to make your communication more effective.

The second part of the book focuses on therapeutic skills. Chapters 4 and 5 describe a range of listening and counselling skills. Chapter 6 is about running groups. Again, the emphasis in these chapters is on developing skills.

The focus of the third part is organizational skills. Senior health professionals (and, increasingly, more junior ones) all have to manage other people. How do you do it? Traditionally, many health professionals have never received training or education in management; they have tended to learn by doing it. Chapter 7 looks at general management skills. Chapter 8 discusses the skills involved in managing meetings and the section closes with a chapter on interview skills.

The final part of the book is more personal. It deals with aspects of self-presentation or what is sometimes called 'impression management'. Chapter 10 identifies a structured approach to improving writing skills. Assertiveness is addressed in Chapter 11 and the book closes with a chapter on a topic that underpins all of the others: self-awareness.

The last section of the book is a Communication Skills Questionnaire which you can use in one or more of the following ways:

- As a self-assessment and self-evaluation instrument before, during and after reading this book;
- As a means of identifying which skills you need to work on further;
- As a basis for discussion in group work.

The book closes with a detailed bibliography of further reading so that the themes in this book can be followed through.

HOW TO USE THE BOOK

The emphasis throughout the book is on two issues:

- The development of practical communication skills;
- The reader's growing awareness of her or his own communication skills.

The aim is always practical. Theory and research are referred to and referenced throughout the text but the reader who wants more detail of any given concept or skill is referred to the detailed bibliography.

You may want to read the book through at one sitting. More likely, though, you will turn to sections or chapters on issues that currently concern you. Each chapter can stand on its own and describes and discusses specific skills. You can easily dip into sections of it.

At the end of each of the four sections, there is a skills checklist. These are to encourage you to reflect further on your own skill levels. They can also encourage discussion or disagreement. As I have noted above, there is no right way in human communication. The point, though, is to become increasingly aware of how *you* communicate and of the effect you have on others when you do.

Finally, a point about language. I have tended to keep it personal throughout the book and refer to 'you' — the reader. I have also referred to the health professional as 'she' and the health care recipient as 'he'. I am aware of the problems of sexism in writing but can find no better compromise at the moment. I have adopted the word 'client' to refer to any health care receiver. Again, I appreciate that some people may prefer the word 'patient' or 'resident' or other descriptor. I feel that the word 'client' is far more straightforward to read than a lengthy 'client/patient/resident' label!

I hope you will find the book useful and enjoy working through the activities. I hope, too, that you will take issue with some (but not all!) of the things I have written. The science and art of human relationships are still fairly new. We have a long way to go before we understand what happens when two or more people meet and talk to each other. In the meantime, as we care for other people, we can try.

PHILIP BURNARD,
Caerphilly, Wales

PART ONE

Educational Skills

INTRODUCTION

Education and training techniques in the health professions are changing. The model that is being adopted increasingly is one that recognizes students as adults. In Part One we explore a range of skills that are important in the education of students. First, the question of teaching skills. If an adult model of education and training is to be used, *facilitation* skills rather than traditional 'telling' techniques will have to be developed. The first chapter explores facilitation and teaching methods.

More and more health care professionals are called upon to speak about their work — either 'in house' or at conferences and workshops. Chapter 2 considers the practical skills that go towards making an effective and professional presentation.

Computers and computing play an increasing part in health care. Every health care professional is likely to come into contact with computers at some stage in their career. At present, we are in an interesting stage of our development, where younger people are likely to know more about the subject than are more senior colleagues. Many health care workers will find that their children know more about computers than they do. The third chapter explores practical aspects of computing as they relate to studying and researching.

Throughout Part One, the emphasis is on education: lifelong education. No health care professional, whatever their discipline can stop studying. We all have to be continual students. There are certain skills that can help us to study, teach and learn more effectively. Part One of this book examines and explores those skills.

1

Teaching skills

Aims of the chapter

The following skills are discussed in this chapter:

- teaching adults
- using experiential learning methods
- planning teaching sessions
- running teaching sessions
- evaluating learning

TEACHING ADULTS

Being an effective communicator often involves teaching and learning. The teaching that is involved is often the teaching of adults. Staff training, professional education, patient or client information-giving: all involve the teaching of adults. In this first section, the principles of adult education are explored and the concept of experiential learning or learning by experience. The chapter goes on from this explanation of experiential learning to consider the planning and execution of facilitation sessions in line with modern educational and therapeutic thought. It closes with the consideration of styles of facilitation. The skills and issues discussed in this chapter are relevant to all health care facilitators whether they are formally designated as such or are those health care professionals who find themselves teaching others or helping them to reflect on their personal experience.

LEARNING FROM EXPERIENCE

People have always learned from experience. We are all made up of huge numbers of personal experiences that shape us and make us the people we are. However, the idea of experiential learning as an educational concept is a relatively recent one. It is, perhaps, far more widely known in the concept of therapy, where the whole subject matter of enterprise is human experience.

Experiential learning was developed out of the work of the American pragmatic philosopher, John Dewey (1916, 1938). Keeton and Associates (1976) described experiential learning as including learning through the process of living and involved work experience, skills developed through hobbies and interests and non-formal educational activities. This approach was reflected in the Further Education Unit project report 'Curriculum Opportunity' which suggested that experiential learning referred to the knowledge and skills acquired through life and work experience and study (F.E.U., 1983). This is particularly pertinent to the work of health professionals. Almost all such professionals develop skills as they work with clients, patients or colleagues.

Pfeiffer and Goodstein (1982) took a different approach by describing an 'experiential learning cycle' which suggested the process of experiential learning. The five stages in their cycle are:

1. Experiencing
2. Publishing (Sharing reactions)
3. Processing (Discussion and dynamics)
4. Generalizing
5. Applying (Planning more effective behaviour)

This cycle not only identified a format for organizing experiential learning but also made reference to the way in which people learn through experience.

Kolb (1984) was more explicit about this learning process in his 'experiential learning model'. Kolb's model included the following stages:

1. Concrete experience;
2. Observations;
3. Formation of abstract concepts and generalizations;
4. Testing implications of and reflections on concepts in new situations.

4

Malcolm Knowles, the American adult educator (Knowles, 1980) took a different approach to the definition of experiential learning. He described the following activities as 'participatory experiential techniques':

- group discussion
- cases
- critical incidents
- simulations
- role play
- skills practice exercises
- field practice exercises
- field projects
- action projects
- laboratory methods
- consultative supervision (coaching)
- demonstrations
- seminars
- work conferences
- counselling
- group therapy
- community development (Knowles, 1980, p. 50)

His list seems so all-inclusive that he seems to have been saying that experiential learning techniques excluded only the lecture method or private, individual study and that experiential learning was synonymous with participant and discovery learning.

Summarizing the position adopted by those writers who devised their definitions of experiential learning from the work of Dewey, would involve noting first the accent on a cycle of events starting with concrete experience. Kolb's and Pfeiffer and Goodstein's cycles were anticipated by Dewey:

> Thinking includes all of these steps, the sense of a problem, the observation of conditions, the formation and rational elaboration of a suggested conclusion and the active experimental testing. (Dewey, 1916, p. 151)

Kolb's notion of transformation of experience and meaning can also be traced back to Dewey. He wrote that:

> In a certain sense every experience should do something to prepare a person for later experiences of a deeper and more

expansive quality. That is the very meaning of growth, continuity, reconstruction of experience. (Dewey, 1938, p. 47)

This was the influence on experiential learning from the Dewey perspective. The accent was on the primacy of personal experience and on reflection as the tool for changing knowledge and meaning.

Boud and Pascoe (1978) summed up what they considered to be the most important characteristics of experiential education thus:

1. The involvement of each individual student in his or her own learning (learning activities need to engage the full attention of a student),
2. The correspondence of the learning activity to the world outside the classroom of the educational institution (the emphasis being on the quality of the experience, not its location),
3. Learner control over the learning experience (learners themselves need to have control over the experience in which they are engaged so that they can integrate it with their own mode of operation in the world and can experience the results of their own decisions). (Boud and Pascoe, 1978, p. 36)

Boud and Pascoes' list seems to sum up the Dewey approach to learning through experience and through responsibility in the learning process.

It was Carl Rogers who offered the clearest definition of what experiential or 'significant' learning might be. He identified these elements of experiential learning:

1. It has the quality of personal involvement,
2. It is self-initiated,
3. It is pervasive,
4. It is evaluated by the learner [rather than by educators],
5. Its essence is meaning. (Rogers, 1972, p. 276)

Whilst the final element ('Its essence is meaning') is rather unclear, Rogers' view of experiential learning was a view of 'personalized' learning, which he contrasted with 'cognitive learning' or the learning of facts and figures that are imposed by educators. Experiential learning, for Rogers, was learning that was self-initiated and in which the learner's interest and motivation was high. He went on to identify 'assumptions relevant to experiential learning':

1. Human beings have a natural potentiality for learning;
2. Significant learning takes place when the subject matter is perceived by the student as having relevance for his own purposes;
3. Much significant learning is acquired through doing;
4. Learning is facilitated when the student participates responsibly in the learning process;
5. Self-initiated learning, involving the whole person of the learner — feelings as well as intellect — is the most pervasive and lasting;
6. Creativity in learning is best facilitated when self-criticism and self-evaluation are primary, and evaluation by others is of secondary importance;
7. The most socially useful learning in the modern world is the learning of the process of learning, a continuing openness to experience, an incorporation into oneself of the process of change. (Rogers, 1972, pp. 278–279)

Here, Rogers not only spells out the nature of experiential learning but adds dimensions about how he perceives human beings. Rogers argues that human beings function at their best when they are allowed to learn for themselves, a theme that will be familiar to most health professionals. In the end, you can probably only rarely *tell* people important things; mostly, they have to learn for themselves.

EXPERIENTIAL LEARNING AND YOUR ROLE AS A HEALTH PROFESSIONAL

Having considered the personal nature of learning as it has been discussed in this section, consider your own learning. Think about the things that you have learned that have *not* involved a teacher or lecturer. It may be possible to discover that most of the important things that we learn, we learn through reflection on our personal experience. If we learn from teachers, then learning occurs most readily, perhaps when they relate what they are teaching to that wealth of personal experience that we carry around with us. As we shall see, the tendency increasingly is to see teachers as 'facilitators of learning' rather than as 'passers on of knowledge'.

Before we go further, however, reflect on this issue of learning from experience. Consider the following list and think about how you learned each of the items on it:

- Relating to others and caring for them;
- Deciding who you like and who you do not;
- Coping with bad news;
- Enjoying your own company;
- Wanting to help other people;
- Liking or not liking yourself;
- Spiritual beliefs or lack of them;
- Sexual identity;
- Personality.

Each of these issues, it is suggested, has more to do with personal experience than it ever does with formal teaching or learning. One of the most important parts of communicating with others is the sharing and developing of personal experience: a recurrent theme throughout this book.

FACILITATION OR TEACHING?

The accent in education in the health professions is changing towards the educational encounter being student-centred rather than teacher-centred and appropriately adult-centred. In this approach, the aim is not to initiate the group participants into particular ways of knowing as Peters (1969) would argue, but to encourage them to think about their own experience and to transform their personal knowledge and skills through the processes of reflection, discussion and action. In the student-centred approach to learning, the health professional educator acts as a facilitator of learning rather than as a teacher.

The notion of 'teacher' suggests one who passes on knowledge to others, who instructs and manages learning for others. The notion of facilitation has other connotations and these are developed in this chapter alongside the practical issues that need to be addressed if the health professional is to function as a facilitator.

Elizabeth King offers the following suggestions about the nature of the facilitator's role:

- They must believe students should make their own decisions and think for themselves.
- They must refrain from assuming an authoritative role and adopt a more facilitative and listening position.
- They must accept diversity of race, sex, values, etc. amongst their students.
- They must be willing to accept all viewpoints unconditionally and not impose their personal values on the students. The ability to entertain alternatives and to negotiate no-lose solutions to problems often leads to group decisions that are more beneficial for both the individual and the group (King, 1984).

In the pages that follow, the term 'facilitator' will be used to denote the health professional who is running a group. That group may be a relatively formal learning group, it may be a therapy group or it may be a relatively informal support group. In principle and in practice, the skills that are involved in helping others to learn from experience turn out to be very similar.

Certain stages in the facilitation process can be described and the facilitator needs to be aware of the processes that can occur in groups. The stages described here are modified from those offered by Malcolm Knowles (1975) in his discussion of facilitating learning groups for adults.

It is arguable that facilitation of learning has more in common with group therapy than it does with teaching. It is recommended that the person who sets out to become a group facilitator gain experience as a member of a number of different sorts of groups before leading one herself. In this way she will not only learn about group processes experientially but she will also see a number of facilitator styles. As Heron (1977a) points out, in the early stages of becoming a facilitator, it is often helpful to base your style on a facilitator that you have seen in action. Later, the style becomes modified in the light of your own experience and you develop your own approach.

The facilitation of learning has applications in many aspects of the health professional's life. It can, for instance, be an important part of learning to be a health professional at all. It can also be used as a means of helping clients or patients to explore their problems. It can also be a method of running support groups and self-help groups. The context, then, is sometimes an educational one, sometimes a therapeutic one and sometimes a supportive one.

STAGES IN THE FACILITATION PROCESS

Setting the learning climate

The first aspect of helping adults to learn or explore themselves is the creation of an atmosphere in which adult learners feel comfortable and thus able to learn. Unlike more formal classroom learning, the student-centred approach asks of the learners that they try things out, take some risks and experiment. If this is to happen at all, it needs to be undertaken in an atmosphere of mutual trust and understanding.

The first aspect of the setting of a learning climate is to ensure that the environment is appropriate. Rows of desks and chairs are reminiscent of earlier schooldays. For the adult learning group it is often better and certainly more egalitarian if learners and facilitator sit together in a closed circle of chairs.

In the early stages of a learning group it is useful if the group members spend time getting to know each other. 'Icebreakers' are sometimes used for this purpose. An icebreaker is a simple group activity that is designed to relax people and allow them to 'let their hair down' a little, thus creating a more relaxed atmosphere, arguably more conducive to learning. An example of an icebreaker is as follows:

> The group stands up and group members mill around the room at will. At a signal from the facilitator, each person stops and introduces herself to the nearest person and shares some personal details. Then each person moves on and at a further signal, stop and greet another person in a similar way. This series of millings and pairings can continue until each group member has met every other, including the facilitator.

Other examples of icebreaking activities can be found elsewhere (Heron, 1973; Burnard, 1990). Their aim is to produce a relaxed atmosphere in which learning can take place and a further gain is that they encourage group participation and the learning of names. They are used by many facilitators in the experiential learning field. Some people, however (including the author), feel more comfortable with a more straightforward form of introduction. The argument, here, is that learners coming to a new learning experience are already apprehensive. Many carry with them memories of past learning experiences which may or may not have been of the 'formal' sort. To introduce those people to icebreakers too early may alienate them before they start. The icebreaker, by its very unorthodoxy, may surprise and upset them. A simpler form of introductory activity is to invite each person in turn to tell the rest of the group the following information:

- their name;
- where they work and their position in the team or organization;
- a few details about themselves that are nothing to do with work.

It is helpful if the facilitator sets the pace for the activity by first introducing herself in this way. A precedent is thus set and the group members have some idea of both what to say and how much to say. The author recalls forgetting this principle when running a learning session in the Netherlands. As a result, each group member talked for about ten minutes apiece and what was intended to be a short introductory activity turned into a lengthy exercise! The golden rule, perhaps, is keep the activity short and sharp and keep the atmosphere light and easy going.

Once group members have begun to get to know each other, either through the use of icebreakers or by the introductory activity described above, the facilitator should deal with domestic issues regarding the group's life. These will include the following:

- when the group will break for refreshments and meal breaks and when it will end;
- a discussion of the aims of the group;
- a discussion of the 'voluntary principle': that learners should decide for themselves whether or not they will take part in any given activity suggested by the facilitator and that no-one should feel pressurized into taking part in any activity either by the facilitator or by the power of group pressure. It is worth pointing out that if a person finds themselves to be the only person sitting out on a particular activity, they should not feel under any further obligation either a) to take part or b) to justify their decision not to take part;
- issues relating to smoking in the group, when smokers are present;
- any other issues identified by either the facilitator or by group members.

11

This early discussion of group 'rules' is an important part of the process of setting the learning climate. The structure engendered by this part of the day helps to allow everyone to feel part of the decision-making and learning process.

Identifying learning resources

In this stage, both learners and facilitator identify the resources for learning that are present within the group. This may be done with the aid of a 'needs/offers' board. A large flip-chart sheet or area of a black or white board is divided into two columns, 'Needs' and 'Offers'. Learners and facilitator(s) then fill this chart in appropriately at the beginning of a course or block of learning. Clearly, this approach cannot be used at the start of the first such course or block, where neither facilitators nor learners will know each other's skills and knowledge bases. After an introductory programme, however, the Needs/Offers board can be used to help determine the content of all future learning encounters.

Once both facilitator(s) and learners have written down their learning needs and what they have to offer the group, each member of that group is then encouraged to put a tick against the items that they feel will most usefully be included in the learning period.

This approach to identifying needs and resources can be used for one-day workshops as well as for week-long study periods. It depends for its success on all members of the learning group being committed to full negotiation of content. Having said that, it would seem reasonable that the facilitator retains the right to add certain 'compulsory' topics to any given programme in line with her perception of what is required to fulfil a particular syllabus.

Planning the learning encounter

Once the learning group's needs and resources have been identified, the group can draw up a learning contract. Types of contract can range from the informally agreed list of topics that will
be used as the basis of discussion and learning during the day or
week, to a planned identification of what will be learned, how
it will be learned and how learning will be evaluated. Such a
contract will draw from the following elements:

- Non-negotiable content drawn from the syllabus
- Wants and offers

The non-negotiable content drawn from the syllabus may serve as a theme for the learning period. On the other hand, it is important that the content drawn from the needs and offers lists are not seen as additions to an already worked-out timetable. The aim is not to offer learners concessions but fully to negotiate a timetable that best suits their wants and needs and yet which also fully prepares them for any examinations and practical work that they will face. The facilitator who helps in the drawing up of this initial learning contract will need to exercise considerable tact and diplomacy in handling the tension between individual and group needs on the one hand and the requirements of the syllabus on the other.

An alternative approach to using learning contracts is for each learner to draw up one for her own use. This may mean that a given group of students does not meet together for the entire period of learning but that some students will be working on their own whilst others are attending lectures, seminars, discussions and practical learning sessions.

Running the learning group

All that remains is for the learning session to progress along the lines that has been negotiated with the group. The facilitator's task is to ensure the smooth running of the group. Variety of method is an important consideration in ensuring that all members get what they need from the learning encounter and the following represents a short list of methods that may be used:

- lectures
- facilitator-led seminars
- student-led seminars
- facilitator-led discussions
- student-led discussions
- leaderless discussions
- experiential learning activities
- buzz groups
- individual learning sessions
- demonstrations

- visits
- invited speakers
- small group project work
- small group discussion followed by large group plenary sessions

It is probably fair to say that most health care trainers will be armed with a variety of teaching and learning strategies (but probably only use a limited number of them) whilst many learners coming to student-centred learning for the first time will tend to imagine that teaching and learning necessarily involves having someone at the front of the group who leads it and does most of the talking. It is helpful if all learners coming to student-centred learning from more traditional approaches are offered a number of sessions on: a) the philosophy of student-centred learning and a rationale for its use; b) the range of teaching/learning methods that are available; and c) practice in a range of teaching/learning methods and feedback on their use.

If student-centred learning is to succeed, it must involve the learners in every respect, including the skilful use of teaching and learning methods. Learning to use these methods is never wasted for they can be used again and again in future learning encounters both within educational establishments and within the clinical setting. In the clinical area, it is clearly inappropriate to use a formal lecture method. It is not uncommon, however, to find mini-classrooms set up in wards and departments which exactly mimic the sorts of traditional learning approaches that the health professionals working there have been subject to. The student-centred approach to learning can encourage the appropriate use of the appropriate learning aid.

Closing the group

Each facilitator will probably develop her own style of closing the group at the end of the day or at the end of a workshop. A traditional way is through summary of what the day has been about. There is an important limitation in this method, which aims at 'closure'. It is asserted that while the facilitator is summing up in this way, she is doing two things that are not particularly helpful. First, she is putting into her own words those of the group members. Second, whilst she is 'closing' in this way, group members are often, silently, closing off their thoughts about the day or the workshop in much the same way that schoolchildren begin to put their books away as soon as a teacher sums up at the end of a lesson. It may be far better to leave the session open-ended and to avoid any sort of summing up.

Alternatively, rather than allowing the day or the workshop to end rather abruptly, the facilitator may choose to use one or more of the following closing and evaluating activities:

Closing activity one

Each person in turn makes a short statement about what they liked least about the day or about the workshop. Each person in turn then makes a short statement about what they liked most about the day or the workshop. No-one has to justify what they say for their statement is taken as a personal evaluation of their feelings and experience.

Closing activity two

Each person in turn makes a short statement about three things that they feel they have learned during the day or the workshop. This may or may not be followed by a discussion on the day's learning.

Closing activity three

The group has an 'unfinished business' session. Group members are encouraged to share any comments they may have about the day or the workshop, either of a positive or negative nature. The rationale for this activity is that such sharing helps to avoid bottled-up feelings and increases a sense of group cohesion.

These, then, are the stages of a typical student-centred learning session and they may be adapted to suit the particular needs of the group and of the facilitator. The final part of the learning encounter may also involve checking through the group's learning contract to see whether or not various aspects have been covered in sufficient depth and whether or not changes need to be made to that contract.

15

FACILITATOR STYLE

Every facilitator needs to make decisions about what to do when working with a particular learning group. What she does in the group may be called her style. Clearly, facilitator styles will vary from person to person according to a variety of variables including previous group experience, teacher training, knowledge and skill levels, personal preferences, personal value systems and personal beliefs about the nature of education. However, it is useful if the facilitator of learning (and particularly the one who is new to facilitation) can consider what decisions she needs to make about her style prior to engaging in facilitation.

Heron (1977a) suggests six dimensions of facilitator style that can help in such decision making. Heron's six dimensions are as follows:

Directive .... Non-directive
Interpretative .... Non-interpretative
Confronting .... Non-confronting
Cathartic .... Non-cathartic
Structuring .... Un-structuring
Disclosing .... Non-disclosing

The facilitator who uses the directive–non-directive dimension will make decisions about how much she intervenes in the process of development of the group. At one end of the dimension, the facilitator may decide to control group discussion almost completely, by asking questions of the group but also by maintaining overall control of what happens in the group. At the other end of the dimension, the facilitator will play a role that is lower in profile and maintain little or no control over what happens in the group, preferring the learners to decide on the way in which the group develops. Whilst the non-directive end of the demension is more student-centred, there are clearly times when facilitator intervention will enable the group to move on and develop further. The skilled facilitator is probably one who can make appropriate decisions about when to be directive and when to remain in the background.

The interpretative–non-interpretative dimension is concerned with the degree to which the facilitator does or does not offer explanations for what happens in the group. Interpretations of group processes can be made from a number of different points of view, including, at least, the following: psychodynamic, sociological, transactional analytical, transpersonal and political. The facilitator who chooses to use interpretation in order to help the learners make sense of what is happening in the group offers a theoretical framework for the learners to work with. The facilitator who offers no interpretation allows the learners to make their own decisions about what is happening and allows them to construct and develop their own theories. The only problem facing the facilitator who never uses an interpretative style of group leadership is that she may have to acknowledge that some groups will neither notice group processes developing nor will they construct theories to account for what happens.

The next dimension is concerned with the degree to which the facilitator does or does not confront the group at any given time in the group's development. At one end of the dimension, the facilitator is very challenging and draws attention to illogicalities and inconsistencies in group arguments. At the other end of the dimension, she sits back and allows members of the group to challenge group debate. Again, as with the other dimensions, it is probably useful if the facilitator can learn to be appropriately confronting and appropriately passive, according to circumstances.

The cathartic–non-cathartic dimension refers to the amount of emotional release that the facilitator allows or seeks in a learning group. It is arguable that during the process of learning counselling and group skills it is helpful if group participants may be allowed to express their feelings as part of the experiential learning process. Sometimes, too, arguments and discussions can be sharpened if participants are allowed to express strong feelings. At other times, however, it is more appropriate that emotional release does not become part of the group process. In a clinical teaching session, for example, or during a ward round, it may not be appropriate for learners to express their feelings directly. It may be more appropriate if that emotion is expressed later during a student–facilitator discussion.

There are specific skills involved in helping people to express emotion. Heron (1977a) argues that in the UK we have developed a 'non-cathartic society', where the norm generally is to bottle up rather than express emotion. He suggests various methods for helping groups to release pent-up emotion and courses in developing cathartic skills are frequently offered by colleges and extra-mural departments of universities.

Emotional release is part of the human condition. It is also frequently a part of the experience of being a patient. If learners never have the opportunity to explore their own feelings then, arguably, they will be less well prepared for handling the emotional release of their patients. This is not to advocate frequent therapy or encounter groups as part of the educational experience but to acknowledge the need for health care facilitators to consider the inclusion of the development of cathartic skills at some point in the health professional education programme.

The structuring–un-structuring dimension is a vital one in terms of student-centred health professional education. The highly structuring facilitator will organize the timetable, decide upon content, carry through the lessons and evaluate the whole procedure. In other words, the structuring facilitator is not particularly student-centred. On the other hand, the facilitator who is totally un-structuring may be one whose learning sessions are an educational 'free for all', with little coherence or development. Again, the answer seems to lie in a sense of balance and an ability to decide when to offer structure to a group and when to allow the group to develop its own.

Heron's final dimension is the disclosing–non-disclosing one. The disclosing facilitator is one who shares with learners much of her own thoughts and feelings, as they emerge. In this sense, she becomes a fellow traveller with the learners. Many years ago, Sidney Jourard (1964) suggested that 'disclosure begets disclosure'. It seems likely that the facilitator who is able to share something of herself with her learners is more likely to encourage them to share something of themselves with the group. Thus the process of education becomes a humanizing process.

On the other hand, there are times when non-disclosure is appropriate. If the facilitator is too disclosing, she may find that she inhibits group participants. Most of us have experienced the person who, at the drop of a hat, tells us his life story, or who too readily discloses his own thoughts or feelings. Almost as important as whether or not we disclose to a group is the decision about when we disclose. As with most things in life, timing is of the utmost importance. Sometimes to hold back and keep our thoughts and feelings to ourselves can encourage quieter members of the group to develop the courage to disclose.

The six dimensions of facilitator style have wide application across many different sorts of learning groups. Facilitators may use them in seminar groups, in organizing discussions, in running support groups and in running learning groups in clinical settings. The dimensions may also be offered to learners as a frame- work for considering their own decisions about running groups. Whenever we engage in a learning encounter, we make certain decisions about how to proceed. The dimensions of facilitator style offered here allow for clear-cut prior decisions to be made. They also allow for 'fine tuning' whilst the group is in progress. The person who has internalized and understood the range of possibilities contained within the six dimensions can quickly change direction whilst working within a group and yet do that with some precision.

SUMMARY OF THE CHAPTER

This chapter has taken a broad view of the process of learning through experience. All health care professionals are concerned with learning: both their own and that of their colleagues. The issues and skills that have been discussed here are relevant to *all* communication skills in the health care professions.

REFERENCES

Boud, D. and Pascoe, J. (1978) *Experiential Learning: Developments in Australian Post-Secondary Education*, Australian Consortium on Experiential Education, Sydney, Australia.

Burnard, P. (1990) *Learning Human Skills: An experiential guide for nurses*, 2nd edn, Heinemann, Oxford.

Dewey, J. (1916) *Democracy and Education*, Free Press, London.

Dewey, J. (1938) *Experience and Education*, Collier Macmillan, London.

F.E.U. (1983) *Curriculum Opportunity: A map of experiential learning in entry requirements to higher and further education award bearing courses*, Further Education Unit, London.

Heron, J. (1973) *Experiential Training Techniques:* Human Potential Research Project, University of Surrey, Guildford, Surrey.

Heron, J. (1977a) *Dimensions of Facilitator Style:* Human Potential Research Project, University of Surrey, Guildford, Surrey.

Heron, J. (1977b) *Behaviour Analysis in Education and Training:* Human Potential Research Project, University of Surrey, Guildford, Surrey.

Jourard, S. (1964) *The Transparent Self*, Van Nostrand, New Jersey.

Keeton, M. and Associates (1976) *Experiential Learning*, Jossey Bass, San Francisco, California.

King, E.C. (1984) *Affective Education in Nursing: A guide to teaching and assessment*, Aspen, Maryland.

Knowles, M. (1975) *Self-Directed Learning*, Cambridge, New York.

Knowles, M.S. (1980) *The Modern Practice of Adult Education*: From pedagogy to andragogy, 2nd edn, Follett, Chicago.

Kolb, D. (1984) *Experiential Learning*, Prentice Hall, Englewood Cliffs, New Jersey.

Peters, R.S. (1969) *The Ethics of Education*, Allen and Unwin, London.

Pfeiffer, J.W. and Goodstein, L.D. (1982) *The 1982 Annual for Facilitators, Trainers and Consultants*, University Associates, San Diego, California.

Rogers, C.R. (1972) The Facilitation of Significant Learning, in M.L. Silberman, J.S. Allender and J.M. Yanoff (eds) *The Psychology of Open Teaching and Learning*, Little Brown, Boston.

2

Presentation skills

Aims of the chapter

The following skills are discussed in this chapter:

- planning a presentation
- using notes and visual aids
- speaking
- taking questions

Have you ever been asked to talk about your work? Many health professionals have. Many too, once over the feeling of being flattered and of having had their self-confidence boosted, go on to worry about how they will cope. This is especially true if they are asked to talk at a conference. Saying 'yes' to a request is the easy part. The more difficult bits are preparing what you have to say and then saying it. In this chapter, the whole process of preparing and giving a presentation are explored.

One thing needs to be clear. Giving a presentation at a meeting or a conference is different from teaching. First of all, the aims are different. The main aim of teaching is to enable and encourage learning. The main aim of a presentation is to offer a clear outline of some particular information. In the process of giving that information, the presenter may be teaching too, but that is not the main aim.

Very often, people go to conferences and presentations to hear very specific information. Often, they are not beginners in a particular field. Rather, they are often co-professionals. On the other hand, it is important to remember when you are asked to give a paper or make a presentation that one of the reasons that you have been asked is that you have information that others do not. You are the expert amongst experts. This can, on the one hand, be an exhilarating thought; on the other, it can be a little worrying. What can help here is *structure*: structure in planning, delivery and follow-up. In the following sections, each of these elements is examined.

PLANNING THE PRESENTATION

First, be clear. Why have you been asked to give a presentation? Is it because you are well known and they just want you at the conference because you are 'you'? If so, it often doesn't matter what your topic is. Indeed, you may be allowed to talk about a topic of your choice. Far more likely, though, is that you have been asked to address a particular set of issues or to report some research findings. First, find out the reason for being asked and be clear about the topic. Find out, too, how long you will be expected to talk, how long you have for questions and whether or not the session will be chaired. If it is, you will be introduced to your audience. If not, you will have to think about how you want to introduce yourself.

Second, to whom will you be talking? To fellow professionals? To a group of learners? If so, at what point in their training or education is that group? What comes before and after your presentation? Also, how many people will be present? Whilst there may not be much difference in making a presentation to 100 or 400, there are important differences between talking to five or 50 people. You need to know in advance how large or small your audience will be.

What will you tell your audience? It is important that you avoid trying to include 'everything' in your presentation. If you are presenting research findings, the important things are the findings themselves. You do not need to go into elaborate background detail, nor (usually) do you need to talk a great deal about sampling procedures. From the audience's point of view, the interesting things are usually what you found in your research.

The other thing that has to be said here is that your presentation of findings must be *interesting*. Bear in mind that you have lived with your work. You have found it fascinating. The task, now, is to inspire others. You can do that if you carefully plan your presentation.

The stages in a presentation, whatever the topic, can be divided up thus:

- Introduction (of self and topic);
- Outline of points to be covered;
- Development of each of the points;
- Summary and brief discussion;
- Inviting questions.

Think carefully about the points that you want to make. Don't make too many of them. Most of us are familiar with the groan that occurs when someone stands up with a prepared flipchart sheet which identifies ten points, after which it is all too clear that the speaker is going to cover each in some detail. Try, if you can, to summarize your work into three or four main headings. Then, whilst the audience has some sort of signposting system through your talk and you have a scaffolding upon which to build your talk, no-one is going to feel overwhelmed.

Once you have identified your three or four main points. Think about how you will introduce the whole talk and how you make it obvious why you are to talk about the points you raise. Remember that your aim is to *inform*. If you have done your research, you will have a reasonable idea of the 'level' of your audience. Once this is established it will usually become clear that you do not have to offer a wide ranging historical introduction to your subject area. Instead, all you need to do is to put your talk into context and wade into your main points.

Think carefully about timing. Whilst this obviously comes with experience of talking, you must try to work out exactly how much you can cover in the time available to you. It is very easy to overestimate how much you can say in a given time. If you stick to the 'three or four points' rule, you are less likely to overrun. Underrunning can also be a problem, although it is a far less important one than overrunning. First, most people are quite happy to sit through a short presentation. Second, you are quite likely to be able to make up time through the question period. It can be argued that the question session is often the most valuable part of the session. On the other hand, if people have come some distance to hear you talk, they may be disappointed if you reach your conclusion after ten minutes of standing up.

One way to judge your timing is to role play your whole presentation with a colleague, a group of colleagues or members of the family. By far the most difficult option (but probably the most useful) is the second one. If you can gather together a group of colleagues to listen and make comments on your proposed presentation, you can learn a lot of tips about how to do it and how to ensure that you neither over- nor underrun. Ask those who listen to you to pay particular attention to the following:

- The way that you start your presentation;
- How you look as you deliver it;
- Your tone of voice and speed of delivery;
- Your use of language and jargon;
- The way you close your presentation.

Listen carefully to what your colleagues or family have to say. This is not always easy. I remember the night before I gave my first paper at an international conference, I was told by a colleague that 'it is a pity you can't do something about your monotonous voice!' I did do something, but I can't guarantee it was the right thing. Throughout the presentation I tried to modulate my voice and probably sounded fairly bizarre. The point, here, is to do the role playing well in advance of your presentation. If they can bear it, have your colleagues listen to you a second time. Be careful, though, that you do not 'wear out' your talk or overrehearse it. Whilst everyone likes a polished performance, no-one likes to have the impression that this is the fourteenth time you have given it.

NOTES

To read from notes or not to? Not to. If at all possible, avoid reading directly from a script or straight from notes. If *you* can read what you have to say, so can your audience. If all you are doing is standing up and reading what you would normally publish in a journal, do the latter. Go away and write your journal paper. Whilst you may not want to do without notes altogether (and few do), you want to try to keep your notes to key issues and an overall outline structure.

The most frequently used method of using notes at a presentation is that of holding a bunch of index cards in your hand, each of which contains notes linked to one of your three or four points. These have advantages and disadvantages. The advantages are that they are easy to hold and to refer to. You can hold your hands up fairly high and this tends to encourage you to speak out to your audience rather than down to your notes. On the other hand, small cards can be dropped. Once dropped, you have the unenviable (but fascinating to the audience in a morbid sort of way) task of picking them up and rearranging them. Just in case, it is best to number your cards with fairly large numbers so that your nervous hands can reorder them in a crisis.

It is usually best to link your cards with your visual presentations. As is noted in the next section, backing up what you say with things that the audience can look at pays distinct dividends. Usually, you can link one card with one visual aid. In this way, you do not have to carry out too many operations at once. Be sure, though, clearly to number both your cards *and* your visual aids. Visual aids can also be dropped or get out of order. If both the card and the aid bear the same number, you are less likely to run into problems.

The alternative to cards is to use a typewritten or computer-generated set of notes. If you use this method, you need to have them typed with double spacing, so that you can read them easily as you glance down. Also, it is useful to make full use of coloured outlining pens. Careful colour coding can show you where you are in relation to your main three or four points: each point can be outlined in a different colour and that colour code can be carried through to your visual aids. The big disadvantage of the typed sheets is that you are likely to be carried away with looking at them.

There is some comfort to be had from holding a large bunch of papers. Often, that comfort takes over and the speaker using them, stares down at them throughout the presentation, sometimes from fear of losing her place. Think, too, about whether or not you staple the sheets together. The advantage of this approach is that you can hold the whole set of pages together, with less fear of dropping them. On the other hand, if you find yourself with a large lectern in front of you, unstapled sheets can more easily be turned over. I have been known to adopt the 'belt and braces' approach and take two sets of notes with me to a conference: one stapled and the other not.

If your confidence really leaves you and you decide that you *must* read from notes, consider the way that you write out those notes. Rather than just typing out a 'script', write out what you say in the way that you say it. The following extract illustrates this. The piece is laid out in such a way that it makes it very clear where you pause and where you take a breath. The idea is that each line contains one phrase. Work carefully through your notes and break them up in this way. This will save you 'fluffing' lines

25

and save you having to re-read what you have said. It must be stressed, however, that reading direct from a paper is the last resort. If you can, avoid it.

Example of the Layout of A Paper to Be Read

Many managers are having to think carefully about how change is
 affecting their organization.
Many are experiencing anxiety about the *rate* of change.
Writers on the topic are not particularly helpful here.
All seem to stress that change is accelerating.
This morning, I want to challenge that view.
The question is:
Is the rate of change *really* increasing?
Think about your own workplace.
What changes have *you* seen?
Major ones?
Or have you experienced a slow trickle of minor changes?

One of the best ways of preparing this sort of paper is on a computer, using a wordprocessor. It is possible, in some programs, to set up 'macros' or short-hand routines that operate 'sentence-busting' functions. Such macros split the whole of your paper up into sentences and put each sentence on a separate line. WordPerfect is one such wordprocessing program. It is possible with this wordprocessor, not only to sentence-bust but also to reverse the process and put the paper back together again. In this way, you are able to prepare the paper that you use for your presentation and the more usual copies of the paper for wider distribution. Be careful, though: splitting the paper into sentences is not *all* that is involved. You also need to go through the piece and underline or accent certain words so that you know exactly when to emphasize your points. Notice, too, that the piece above is not strictly grammatical. You may want to consider the use of rhetorical questions that 'sound' right, when you speak but would not normally be acceptable in a written paper. Again, this is further fuel for the argument that you should try to avoid reading directly from a script. On the other hand, if you are giving a lot of very detailed information and that information must be exactly right, then reading may be your only option. Consider, for example, newsreaders on the television. No-one would expect them to extemporize with the help of cue cards.

VISUAL AIDS

Back up what you say with a visual aid. Almost all presentations can be more interesting if they are also offered visually. On the other hand, be wary of overusing such aids. If too many are used, the audience can become distracted by waiting to see what else happens in your 'performance' and it loses track of what you are saying.

Why use visual aids at all? A number of important reasons can be identified:

- Some people absorb information far more easily in a visual mode than they do in an aural one,
- The visual aid adds interest to what you are saying,
- Some things can only be conveyed visually (imagine trying to say what a magnified snowflake looks like),
- A visual aid takes attention off of the speaker and allows him or her to breathe more easily,
- People like them.

The key issues that apply to all visual aids are: a) keep them simple and uncluttered and b) keep them few in number. First, it is important that visual presentations do not contain hundreds of words and that the audience does not have to spend the next five minutes reading. Remember that all the time the audience is reading your visual aid, it is not listening to you. This means that some of your presentation will be lost. If it is, your audience may be unable, or unwilling, to catch up. Second, nothing is more daunting than the realization that a speaker has 20 visual aids to work through. Keep them short and keep them few in number. Finally, remember that once a visual aid has been referred to and seen, it is important to remove it from the audience's eyes.

Four main sorts of visual aids for presentations can be identified:

- overhead transparencies
- flipcharts
- slides
- video tapes

Overhead transparencies are probably known to everyone who has been involved in teaching or learning. They are fairly easy to

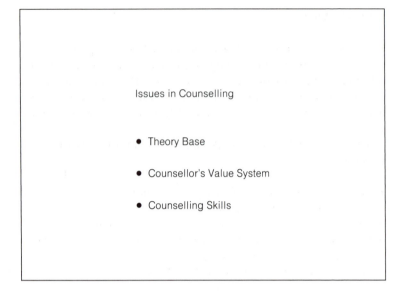

Figure 2.1   Example of a prepared overhead acetate sheet

prepare and can quickly convey a lot of information. What is not always appreciated is how they should be prepared. It is not uncommon to see handwritten transparencies. Far better are those prepared with a graphics package on a computer. This is as true for transparencies that contain only words as it is for those which are pictorial. Both sorts can first be drawn or typed using a program such as Harvard Graphics or Applause. Once the detail has been produced with such a program, the results can be printed out onto paper and then transferred to the acetate sheet via a photocopier. The result is nearly always more professional than is the case with a handwritten or handdrawn sheet. If such graphics programs are not available, another approach is to type words onto paper, enlarge the output with a photocopier and then transfer the enlarged images onto the acetate. As a rule, the less that is contained on an acetate sheet, the better. Do not type line after line. Instead, either use a series of sheets or depend upon one or two pithy lines. Figure 2.1 illustrates an example of what may go onto a single sheet. As a rule, simplicity is the keynote in overhead projector sheets. Coloured sheets may be used to add interest or to differentiate between different issues but, again, be careful. It is easy to find that your audience gets caught up with the *son et lumière* than with what you have to say.

The flipchart sheet has become popular over the last ten years. Flipcharts are giant drawing pads on which the presenter either has prepared sheets of information or on which he or she writes during the presentation. Bear in mind that many people are used to the use of flipcharts in small group work in which participants 'brainstorm' ideas onto such sheets. The very presence of a flipchart pad and easel may have some of the audience ready to (and perhaps anxious about) breaking into groups to work with their colleagues.

Similar rules about the preparation of acetate sheets apply to the preparation of flipchart presentations. Because the size of a flipchart pad is so large, it is always tempting to overfill each sheet. Resist this. Keep to a brief message, as with acetate sheets. The items listed in Figure 2.1 could easily be transferred to a flipchart pad, without addition of other material.

Flip chart sheets must necessarily be hand drawn (although, in extreme circumstances, it may be possible to use Letraset or similar graphical lettering products). They have, however, one big advantage over overhead projector sheets. The bulb in an overhead projector is a fragile thing. Murphy's law dictates that the bulb will blow just as you come to your first acetate sheet and when you are feeling most vulnerable. If you are nervous of this happening and you are not talking to a very large group, you may choose to use a flipchart.

If you prepare your sheets before the conference, consider leaving the first white sheet of the pad blank, then you need only disclose what is written on each of your sheets once you have started talking. If you are allowed free use of the pad, you may want to leave a blank sheet between written sheets too. In this way, you can take a break between each of the sheets, rather in the way that you might turn the overhead projector off between acetates.

If you are going to write on the pad as you talk, be sure that your writing is neat enough to be read. It does not have to be particularly large. Usually, letters of about 1.5″ in height can easily be read by most of a medium-sized audience. Resist the temptation to doodle on the pad, or to write down unconnected words or diagrams. Write neatly and clearly and express only one or two ideas on each sheet. If you need to, you can tear off each sheet and 'Bluetack' it up on a wall. This does, however, take confidence. If you are nervous, it is very easy flamboyantly to rip straight through the middle of your sheet as you tear it off.

An alternative to the flipchart is the traditional black- or (less traditional) whiteboard. Both have fallen into disuse as an aid during presentations and conferences, perhaps because of their classroom connotations. If you do use either of them, practise first. Both take experience to use effectively. It is easy, for instance, to find yourself talking *to* a whiteboard. It is also easy to break chalk. Finally, it is not uncommon for both chalk and whiteboard pens to run out at a critical moment. Perhaps, after all, it is for these reasons that such visual aids are rarely seen today.

Slides are yet another way of displaying parts of a presentation graphically. Whilst they are easily the most interesting format of all of the visual aids mentioned so far, they also have a variety of drawbacks. First, they are expensive to produce and difficult to produce well. It is not sufficient to be a keen amateur if you want to produce really effective slides: such productions can make the whole presentation look amateurish. If you do use slides, have them professionally produced.

Another drawback to the use of slides is that so much can (and often does) go wrong. First, the slide projector can break down, either before or during your presentation. Second, because of nerves, it is very easy to put slides into the slide carousel upside-down or in the wrong order. This is usually guarded against if you have slides professionally made for presentation. Then, the 'right side up' is usually marked on each slide. This does not, however, stop you putting them into the carousel in the wrong order. Also, if you show slides, you usually have to dim the lights. This takes the spotlight off you (which you may think is a good thing). On the other hand, once you are out of the limelight, the audience may forget you and pay more attention to your slides, becoming impatient to see the next one.

Having said all that, well-produced slide packages can easily outshine all other forms of visual aid for impact on the audience. Even slides with lettering on (used in the place of overhead projector acetates) add an air of authority to the presentation. Graphs, bar charts and histograms always look more professional if they are shown on slides. The usual rule applies though: put very little on each slide. This may be slightly more expensive but it is much better than presenting slides covered in words, figures or images.

Think carefully about the visual aids that you choose. Try to go to other people's presentations and see what worked best for them. Then choose your own aids. You may or may not want to use more than one sort of aid: slides and a flip chart, for example. Do avoid too much visual razzmatazz. As noted earlier, it is possible for the audience to become so impressed with the 'show' that they stop paying attention to you or your presentation.

SPEAKING

When you are speaking to an audience, you want to communicate with as many members of it as possible. Certain straightforward rules apply here. First, be careful about your posture. Stand up straight, try not to wander around in front of those to whom you are speaking and keep an eye on your breathing. It is useful to begin the whole presentation by taking one or two deep breaths before you start. This nearly always seems to you as though you are standing silent for about 15 minutes. To the audience, however, it is a chance really to focus their thoughts on you and to settle down in their seats.

A common error when speaking in public is to focus eye contact and attention on one person. This may be due to some well-meaning but often misconstrued advice that you should 'find someone in the audience and speak to them'. There is nothing worse than being the person to whom the speaker is speaking. Pay attention to your eye contact. Try to make regular sweeps of the audience, punctuated by picking out various members of the assembly to address certain parts of your talk to. Avoid looking down at your notes as much as possible. It is here that having cards, rather than a typed script, can really pay off. The fact that you only have a small card in your hand means that your eye is not so easily drawn to it.

Be careful of the hand gestures that you make. It is easy to be carried away in your talk and forget that your hands are 'talking for you'. Make gestures mean something. If necessary (and this is difficult) practise some gestures in front of a mirror or in front of a colleague. Notice what works and what does not. Watch commentators on the television and see what gestures they use. Watch politicians, too, for they are often masters and mistresses of effective gesture.

Finally, keep an eye on all aspects of your voice. Important, here, are the tone, volume and pitch. It is not recommended that you try to change your accent if you are not happy with it but you can practise developing the tone of your voice. As a general rule, the more relaxed you are, the more likely it is that your tone will be deeper and more full. If you are very nervous, your voice is likely to become thinner. Again, remember the deep breaths just before you start and if you get very nervous, practise some deep breathing before your whole presentation.

Check the volume of your voice before you start. One way of doing this is to arrive a little early and ask someone to sit at the back of the room. Then ask them if they can hear you clearly. If you cannot do this, it is sometimes helpful to ask, at the beginning of your presentation, if everyone can hear you, especially at the back. The problem with this approach is that even if people can hear you, they are sometimes loath to call out the fact.

Prior role play can help you assess the best pitch of your voice. Is your voice naturally mellifluous or do you tend to drone a little? If you are prone to monotony in your speaking, practise a few changes of down and add a few 'ups and downs'. In this respect, you will have to become a little like an actor. Indeed, it could be argued that part of the success of being an effective speaker is being able to act the part. If you look and sound the part, you probably *are* the part. Or as Kurt Vonnegut wrote in one of his novels (Vonnegut, 1969) 'We are what we pretend to be. So take care *what* you pretend to be.'

TAKING QUESTIONS

Once you have given your talk or presentation, there will often be a space for you to take questions. If the conference or talk is being chaired, the chairperson will deal with questions from the floor. If not, you have to manage them yourself. It is helpful (and gives you a little time to adjust to the person asking the question) if you suggest that each person introduces themself by name and occupation before they ask their question. This gives you a little more control over your audience. After all, there are lots of them and only one of you. If there are lots of requests to ask questions, indicate (and remember) who you will take questions from. For example, you may say: 'I'll take the lady at the back's question first, and then one from the gentleman on the right.' *Do* keep track. People don't like to feel that they have been left out. Also, limit questions, initially, to one per person. This not only spreads out the questions, but it also saves your becoming embroiled in detailed discussions with one person. Particularly, look out for the following 'danger' questions:

- Questions that seek to show you up. If you have one of these, there are at least two ways of dealing with it. First, you answer it as best you can and say 'does that deal with your point?' or you deflect the question by saying something like 'that's an interesting point: perhaps we could discuss that after the meeting'. Don't feel that you have to answer every question: listen to how politicians avoid most questions!
- Questions that are five questions rolled into one. Here, you need to be skilful at unpacking. You may want to dissect out the various issues or you may choose to answer just the first question by saying: 'I think I'll just deal with the first point you raise . . .'
- Questions from someone who claims to be a 'friend'. This approach is usually heralded by the person calling you by your first name and by their saying: 'We talked some time ago, in York, about some of the things you have described this morning . . .' This is a particularly awkward way of being presented with a question. Sometimes the question is a 'barbed' one or one that seeks to put you into a difficult light. Try not to be thrown by the immediate intimacy of the questioner's approach and answer the question with a level approach. Avoid sharing the supposed intimacy. Sometimes, of course, you will suddenly be asked a question by someone that you really *do* know. A couple of years ago, I found myself being asked a question by a cousin who I had not seen for about a decade. Again, here you need to take a deep breath, avoid public reminiscences and answer the question as clearly as you can.

Bear in mind that most people are on your side. They are also genuinely interested in what you have to say — they would not have come to the talk or conference if that wasn't the case. If you can, take the fact that you have been asked to speak as a compliment. Enjoy yourself if you can but don't get carried away. Keep an eye on the clock or put your watch down in front of you and stick to a firm schedule. Then, stand back, and let them know that you've arrived!

SUMMARY OF THE CHAPTER

This chapter has examined a number of aspects of presenting your work to an audience. It has described the importance of preparation and structure. It has also discussed some of the visual aids that you may want to use to illustrate your talk. Finally, it has discussed some of the personal issues involved in the 'presentation of self'. At a conference or talk, you are doing just that — you are selling yourself. Do it well.

REFERENCES

Vonnegut, K. (1969) *Mother Night*, Gollancz, London.

3

Computing skills

Aims of the chapter

The following issues are discussed in this chapter:

- buying a computer
- using a computer
- wordprocessing
- spreadsheets
- graphics
- databases

You can't go far without encountering computers in one form or another. The present generation of children and students are growing up completely computer literate. Older health professionals may be struggling to come to terms with using computers. Either way, many people arrive at the point where they have to decide whether or not to buy one. If they do decide to buy one, they have next to think about what sort and about what software to buy. In this chapter, we explore aspects of buying and working with home computers. Many of the issues in this chapter will also apply to using computers at work in both clinical and community settings.

BUYING A COMPUTER

Why buy a computer at all? Many people are finding that they are useful for a range of applications in the home (Burnard, 1990). The most usual reason for buying one, as far as health professionals are concerned, is for completing course work towards further education or degree studies or for research work.

Other obvious applications in the health professional and home context are:

- for the preparation of teaching material;
- for the keeping of notes;
- for the maintenance of bibliographies and book lists;
- for doing accounts;
- for keeping address and contact lists.

What computer should you buy? Computer hardware (the keyboard, monitor and computing unit itself) is changing rapidly. It is also dropping in price. Any specific advice about particular models of computer would be out of place here. Certain general suggestions may be made. A computer for use in the home, that is not going to age too quickly, should fulfil most and perhaps all of the following criteria:

- It should be IBM compatible. IBM set a certain standard for computing equipment at the end of the 1980s. Whilst many computers are 'IBM clones' and whilst it is not necessary to buy a genuine IBM machine, it is essential that the computer that you buy is fully compatible with IBM machines,
- It should have a hard disc. A hard (as opposed to a floppy) disc is capable of storing vast amounts of data. Whilst larger capacity floppy discs are being developed, hard discs currently allow for the storage of 20, 40, 70, 100, 300 mb of data and above. The hard disc also allows you to store all of your programs inside the computer and saves you having to find discs and load up programs from outside.
- It should be expandable. Many computers have expansion slots inside them which allow for upgrading in line with current technological developments. Some of the cheaper and smaller ones do not. It is not necessary to keep changing hardware to keep up with every development. On the other hand, if you do not keep up with some of the main developments, you may find that you can no longer find software to work with your computer as it gets older.
- It should have a monitor and keyboard that suit you. On the monitor issue, many feel that a black and white screen is ideal for wordprocessing. On the other hand, some feel that a

colour screen gives them more flexibility. Yet others prefer a large size screen that allow you to see and work on a whole A4 page of print at a time. Obviously, larger screens also cost more and are non-standard. Similarly, the 'feel' of a keyboard is the subject of much debate. Some prefer a keyboard that reminds them of a typewriter and 'clicks' when the keys are pressed. Others prefer a quieter keyboard. It is recommended that you try typing on a range of keyboards before you choose yours. This is one of the problems when buying computers through the post. Unless you have had experience of the model that you order, you will not be able to try out the keyboard before you buy.

- It should have sufficient RAM (random access memory) to allow you to use modern programs. As computers develop, so the random access memory requirements grow. Until fairly recently, a computer that had 640 k of memory was thought to be adequate. Then the usual figure was 1 mgb. Now it is not uncommon to find machines with 4–8 mgb fitted as standard. If you cannot afford to buy a computer with much RAM fitted as standard, make sure that you can expand the memory at a later date.

Where should you buy a computer? It is sometimes tempting to walk into high street branches of electrical stores and wander round their computer departments trying to decide what you should buy. This is fine if you know what you are looking for but the assistants in such shops are rarely computer experts. It is probably better to enlist the help of a computer expert at work — someone who knows about your own work and your own computing needs.

Most health organizations have one or two resident computer bores — you shouldn't have to look far. Second, become familiar with the computers that you have at work. Learn about them, their capacities and their costs. Then get to know the computer magazines and begin to compare prices. Often, the process of buying through the post can be an excellent way of obtaining a good computer at a fair price. The obvious limitation is that you must know what sort of computer you want. Also, make sure that the firm that you buy it from offers you after-sales service.

Whilst most computers are fairly reliable and have relatively few moving parts to break down, it is important that you can get help on the spot when you need it. Watch out for the companies that insist on a 'back to base' warranty. This means that if your computer breaks down at home, you are responsible for returning it to the company.

There is never a right time to buy a computer. It seems to be a fact of life that just as you get your first computer, you come to realize that it is already out of date. This is a reflection on the rapid development of the computing industry that shows no sign of levelling off. You just have to live with it.

Once you have bought your computer (or better still, before you buy it) learn to type. It is surprising how many people still use the 'hunt and peck' approach to the keyboard and continue to type with two fingers. Part of developing keyboard skills is learning to type. Two approaches are possible here. On the one hand it is practical to attend evening classes in typing or a weekend intensive workshop. On the other hand, there are now many software packages that allow you to develop typing skills at the keyboard. Such programs offer a graded and timed approach to learning how to type and are a cost-effective and time-economical way of advancing keyboard skills.

USING A COMPUTER

Get into the habit of working in a consistent way with your computer. If you have a hard disc, make sure that you organize your files on it in a logical way. With the large amounts of space available on such a disc, it is quite easy to lose files if you do not organize them into directories and subdirectories. The manuals that come with your computer when you buy it will tell you how to do this.

The one golden rule of computing is to make frequent backups of your work. That is to say that you always have more than one copy of every file that you work on. Then, if a file gets lost, destroyed or 'corrupted' in some way, your work has not been lost. This rule is particularly important if you have a hard disc. It is easy to adopt the habit of believing that hard discs are reliable and not subject to breakdown. Generally, this is true. The point is, though, that hard discs have a finite life. At some point, they all do break down. If this happens and you have not made backups of your work, you work is lost. Make backups of all the writing that you do and of any new data files that you work on. If, for example, you add references to your bibliographic database (see below), make sure that you back up the database onto another disc.

WORDPROCESSING

The wordprocessor is probably the most frequently used program in any home or office computer. What can it do? Essentially, it allows you to edit and re-edit your work without having to retype everything that you have written. Compare this with typewriting. If you use a typewriter and make a mistake, you have two options:

- You use a correction paper or fluid and risk making a mess of the pager or,
- You retype the whole page.

With a wordprocessor, neither of these options is necessary. If you make a mistake, if you want to re-order paragraphs or change the text completely, you merely move back up the screen and make the changes. Only when you are completely happy with what you have written do you print out your final 'hard' copy. Wordprocessors vary immensely in their complexity. As with all things, you tend to get what you pay for — the more fully featured programs tend to be very expensive. Check before you buy one that a) you need all the features on offer and b) you will be able to learn how to use it fairly easily. Like other skills, wordprocessing takes practice. It is not like sitting down at a typewriter and beginning to type. With a wordprocessing program you need to invest some time in learning how to use it. Such learning is repaid by cleaner pages, better organized work and the knowledge that you are no longer frightened of computers. Some of the important features to look for in a wordprocessor are these:

- ability to move text easily;
- a spellchecking routine;
- a feature for wordcounting;
- the ability to work with more than one document at once;
- the ability to insert page numbers.

As you become more proficient at wordprocessing you may want to move up to a more comprehensive program, especially if you do a lot of business, academic or creative writing. Other, more advanced features include:

- an indexing facility;
- the ability to work with graphics, diagrams and boxes;
- a thesaurus facility;
- a function for pulling together a number of files;
- macros or the ability to enter a string of commands with a single key stroke.

SPREADSHEETS

A spreadsheet program allows you to develop a huge 'rows and columns' chart on your computer. It does more than this: it also allows you to undertake a whole range of calculations on each or on a selection of the rows and columns. In some ways it is like a computerized and automated accounts book. On the other hand, it can also do far more than just compute rows and columns. It can be used for at least the following functions:

- storing addresses;
- compiling bibliographies and reference lists;
- drawing 'word illustrations' in column format.

GRAPHICS

Graphics packages allow you to illustrate and generally 'dress up' your work. A top commercial package will help you to do the following:

- generate graphs, histograms and pie charts;
- use 'clip art' to illustrate newsletters and projects;
- make slide presentations;
- generate charts for use as overhead projections in teaching;
- draw organization charts.

A good graphics program can help to make your work look more professional and can help you to communicate your thoughts through iconic representation. A basic rule applies here, though: keep it simple. Graphics programs can generate very complicated illustrations and diagrams. It is easy to get carried away with what they can do. Generally communication is much clearer if you stick to simple charts and representations.

DATABASES

After the wordprocessor, the database program is probably one of the most useful for the student, teacher and practitioner in the health professions. Essentially, a database program helps you to store information in a readily retrievable format. The obvious use of a database in this context is for storing references and bibliographies. Databases can also be used for storing other sorts of information, from simple names and address lists through to patient records. Clearly, if the latter are being kept, it is important to see that you comply with the Data Protection Act. Database programs will usually allow you to:

- index your information in various ways;
- print reports of selected information;
- transfer information from the database to other programs;
- allow 'mail-merging' or the generation of multiple letters addressed to different people.

Again, the keyword is simplicity. Commercial database programs are very powerful and often quite difficult to learn to use. If your aim is to keep track of a number of bibliographies, try one of the simpler database programs. Alternatively, you may decide merely to keep your bibliographies as files within your wordprocessor. There are a number of advantages to this approach. First, you can very readily transfer information from the data file to the one you are working in. Second, you do not have to close down one program in order to access your lists of references. Third, you do not have to learn another program. On the other hand, a database program will be much faster and much more versatile if you have bibliographies that run into hundreds of references. I used a file in my wordprocessor to list all my references until the number reached about 500. Then I switched to using a database for them and found the increase in speed and accessibility paid off considerably.

Some people never use databases for storing references and prefer to stick to a card file. The argument is usually that it is just as quick to flip through a box of cards for a reference as it is to start up the computer and fire up the database program. This is fine if the card file is not too big. The point about a database program is that it can let you make selective searches of your references and can allow you to print them out. For example, it can let you pull out all the references that you have on counselling or all those by a particular author and about a specific topic. It can show you all of the papers written on a particular topic after or before a certain data and so on.

COMMERCIAL SOFTWARE

Commercial software refers to the programs that are sold on the open market and produced by software companies. Many of the best known programs are very expensive to buy. On the other hand, they are nearly always very reliable and trustworthy. They also come with very detailed handbooks about their use. If you buy commercial software, only you are allowed to use it. You cannot make copies of it for your colleagues and friends.

The example of a book is useful here. If you buy a book, you can lend it to another person and whilst they have it, you cannot read it. What you must not do is photocopy that book. Commercial software usually works on a similar principle. Once you have bought a copy of a program, it must only be used by one person at a time and copies must not be made for distribution to others. The only exception to this general rule is that most companies allow you to make a backup copy of the program in case the original discs are damaged. Figure 3.1 offers examples of some commercial programs.

SHAREWARE

Shareware has a unique marketing strategy. A shareware program is distributed free of charge (although a charge is usually made for the discs and the handling.) The idea is that you first try the program and then, if you like it, you send away a registration fee to use the program. In the first instance, you usually have between 30 and 90 days to try out the program before you register it. Further, during this time, you are encouraged to make copies of the program for your colleagues and friends. Then, the

Commercial Wordprocessing Programs
WordPerfect
WordStar
Word
Commercial Spreadsheet Programs
1–2–3
Quattro
VisiCalc
Commercial Database Programs
dbase
Paradox
FoxPro

Figure 3.1　Examples of commercial software programs

same principles apply: they are allowed to try out the program and then send off to become registered users if they find it useful.

The advantages of the shareware approach are many for the home PC user. First, he or she has a chance to try the program before making a financial commitment to it. Second, the registration fees for shareware are considerably cheaper than the purchase price of copies of most commercial programs. Also, the quality of shareware programs is improving all the time and some of the best are easily the equal of commercial software. Finally, shareware offers you the easy approach to learning more about computer programs and allows you to explore a variety of methods of working with data that may not have been possible if you had to rely on buying commercial packages. Figure 3.2 illustrates some of the shareware programs that are available. The names and addresses of shareware distributors are available in any of the monthly computer magazines. Such magazine offers include one or two shareware programs on a free disc attached to the front cover.

Shareware is not free. The idea, as we noted above, is to try out the program, decide if you like it and then pay for it. If you decide not to use the program then you simply give the discs to

Shareware Wordprocessing Programs
Galaxy
PC Type
Mindreader
Shareware Spreadsheet Programs
As Easy As
PC Calc
Mipscalc Plus
Shareware Database Programs
PC File
Zephyr
File Express

Figure 3.2 Examples of Shareware software programs

another person or format the discs for use with other files. The only free programs are those available in the public domain. These public domain programs are often distributed by the same people that handle shareware although it is often not made clear in their catalogues what is shareware and what is public domain.

There are various other sorts of programs available that are useful to the health professional. Some of them are commercial programs but a good many are available as shareware. A short list of these would include:

- statistical packages,
- personal organizers and diaries,
- accounting packages,
- computer aided drawing programs,
- desktop publishing programs,
- educational programs,
- aids to learning about computing,
- programs that allow you to communicate with other computers.

As your knowledge and use of computers increases and as computing equipment becomes cheaper, you may want to consider buying a modem. A modem allows you to send computer files down a standard telephone line to another computer. It also allows you to contact other computer users through 'bulletin boards' or computerized message stations. A considerable amount of shareware is available through this means and also an amount of public domain or free software.

A modem can also aid communication between where you work and where you live. You may choose, for example, to work at home on certain days and to send in your work via the modem. This is of particular value to those who engage in writing reports and printed matter.

SUMMARY OF THE CHAPTER

This chapter has considered a range of issues relating to computers as a means of communication in the health care setting. In the end, we all have to use them. To learn about them now is an investment. Who knows, you might learn to love them.

REFERENCES

Burnard, P. (1990) So you think you need a computer?, *The Professional Nurse*, **6**, no. 2, 119–20.

Skills Check: Part One

Sit quietly and reflect on the skills that have been discussed in this section. How many of them are applicable in your health care setting? To what degree do you feel that you have had training in those that are applicable?

Now ask yourself the following questions:

- What do I need to do to enhance my skills in the area of education?
- How effective am I as a teacher?
- What are my presentational skills like?
- If I were asked to make a presentation tomorrow, what would I have to do now?
- Do I have the skills I need in computing?
- Do I use computers effectively?

PART TWO

Therapeutic Skills

INTRODUCTION

All health professionals have a therapeutic role. The process of helping to care for others means that we engage in talking, counselling or advising as part of our everyday work. Part Two examines some of the specific skills that can be called 'therapeutic'.

Chapter 4 explores that most important of all skills — the skill of listening and paying attention to another person. This skill, like any other, can be learned and can be improved upon. The point of this chapter is to reflect on the elements that go to improve listening and to identify various blocks to listening. We can all learn to listen better.

Counselling has been variously defined. Some see it as part of a managerial function. Others see it almost exclusively as having to do with psychotherapy. Chapter 5 identifies a range of aspects of counselling in health care and considers some of the specific skills of counselling.

Chapter 6 focuses on group work. How do you organize and facilitate groups? What are the stages that most groups go through? The aim of this chapter is to identify the practical and theoretical issues that need to be addressed by anyone planning to set up and run a therapeutic group. The skills involved may also be useful to those running other sorts of groups: support groups, case conferences, management groups and so on. This section, then, considers a range of *therapeutic* communication skills. They link with the educational ones identified in Part One but also stand on their own.

4

Listening skills

Aims of the chapter

The following skills are discussed in this chapter:

- giving attention
- listening
- the behavioural aspects of listening
- blocks to effective listening

Listening and attending are by far the most important aspects of being a health care professional. Everyone needs to be listened to. Unfortunately, most of us feel that we are obliged to talk! Unfortunately, too, it is 'overtalking' by the health care professional that is least productive. If we can train ourselves to give our full attention and really listen to the other person, we can do much to help them. First, we need to discriminate between the two processes, attending and listening.

ATTENDING

Attending is the act of truly focusing on the other person. It involves consciously making ourselves aware of what the other person is saying and of what they are trying to communicate to us. Figure 4.1 demonstrates three hypothetical zones of attention. The zones may help further to clarify this concept of attending and has implications for improving the quality of attention offered to the client.

Zone one in Figure 4.1 represents the zone of having our attention fully focused 'outside' of ourselves and on the environ-

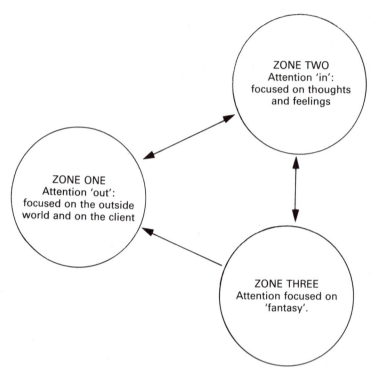

Figure 4.1 Three possible zones of attention

ment around us or, in the context of counselling, on the client. When we have our attention fully focused 'out' in this way, we are fully aware of the other person and not distracted by our own thoughts and feelings.

There are some simple activities, borrowed from meditation practice, that can help and enhance our ability to offer this sort of attention. Here is a particularly straightforward one. Stop reading this book for a moment and allow your attention to focus on an object in the room that you are in: it may be a clock, or a picture or a piece of furniture — anything. Focus your attention on the object and notice every aspect of it: its shape, its colour, its size and so forth. Continue to do this for at least one minute. Notice as you do this, how your attention becomes fully absorbed by the object. You have focused your attention 'out'. Then discontinue your close observation. Notice what is going on in your mind. What are your thoughts and feelings at the moment? When you do this, you shift your attention to zone two: the 'internal' domain of thoughts and feelings. Now shift the focus of your attention out again and onto another object. Study every aspect of it for about a minute. Notice, as you do this, how it is possible consciously to shift the focus of your attention in this way. You can will yourself to focus your attention outside of yourself. Practise at this conscious process will improve your ability to focus attention fully outside of yourself and onto the client.

If we are to pay close attention to every aspect of the client, it is important to be able to move freely between zones one and two. In practice, what probably happens in a counselling session is that we spend some time in zone one, paying full attention to the client, and then we shuttle back into zone two and notice our reactions, feelings and beliefs about what they are saying, before we shift our attention back out. The important thing is that we learn to gain control over this process. It is no longer a haphazard, hit-and-miss affair but we can learn to focus attention with some precision. It is not until we train ourselves consciously to focus attention 'out' in this way that we can really notice what the other person is saying and doing.

Zone three in the diagram involves fantasy — ideas and beliefs that we have that bear no direct relation to what is going on at the moment but concerns what we think or believe is going on. When we listen to another person, it is quite possible to think and believe all sorts of things about them. We may, for example, think ' I know what he's really trying to tell me. He's trying to say that he doesn't want to go back to work, only he won't admit it — even to himself!'

When we engage in this sort of 'internal dialogue' we are working within the domain of fantasy. We cannot know other things about people, unless we ask them, or as Epting puts it: 'if you want to know what another person is about, ask them, they might just tell you!' (Epting, 1984). We often think that we do know what other people think or feel, without checking with that person first. If we do this, it is because we are focusing on the zone of fantasy; we are engaged in the processes of attribution or interpretation. The problem with these sorts of processes is that, if they are wrong, we stand to develop a very distorted picture of the other person. Our assumptions naturally lead us to other assumptions and if we begin to ask questions directly generated by those assumptions, our counselling will lack clarity and our client will end up very confused.

A useful rule, then, is that if we find ourselves within the domain of fantasy and we are 'inventing' things about the person in front of us, we stop and if necessary check those inventions with the client to test the validity of them. If the client confirms them, all well and good — we have intuitively picked up something about the client that he was, perhaps, not consciously or overtly telling us. If, on the other hand, we are wrong, it is probably best to abandon the fantasy altogether. The fantasy, invention or assumption probably tells us more about our own mental make-up than it does about that of our client. In fact, these wrong assumptions can serve to help us gain more self-awareness. In noticing the wrong assumptions we make about others, we can reflect on what those assumptions tell us about ourselves.

Awareness of focus of attention and its shift between the three zones has implications for all aspects of counselling. The health care professional who is able to keep attention directed out for long periods is likely to be more observant and more accurate than the health care professional who is not. The health care professional who can discriminate between the zone of thinking and the zone of fantasy is less likely to jump to conclusions about their observations or to make value-judgements based on interpretation rather than on fact.

What is being suggested here is that we learn to focus directly on the other person (zone one) with occasional moves to the domain of our own thoughts and feelings (zone two) but that we learn, also, to attempt to avoid the domain of fantasy (zone three). It is almost as though we learn to meet the client as a 'blank slate': we know little about them until they tell us who they are. To work in this way in counselling is, almost paradoxically, a much more empathic way of working. We learn rapidly not to assume things about the other person but to listen to them and to check out any hunches or intuitions we may have about them.

Being able to focus on zone one and have our attention, focusing out has other advantages. In focusing in this way, we can learn to maintain the 'therapeutic distance' referred to in a previous chapter. We can learn to distinguish clearly between the client's problems and our own. It is only when we become mixed up by having our attention partly focused on the client, partly on our own thoughts and feelings and partly on our fantasies and interpretations, that we begin to be confused about what the client is telling us and what we are 'saying to ourselves'. We easily confuse our own problems with those of the client.

Second, we can use the concept of the three domains of attention to develop self-awareness. By noticing the times when we have great difficulty in focusing attention 'out', we can learn to notice points of stress and difficulty in our own lives. Typically, we will find it difficult to focus attention out when we are tired, under pressure or emotionally distressed. The lack of attention that we experience can come to serve as a signal that we need to stop and take stock of our own life situation. Further, by allowing ourselves consciously to focus 'in' on zones two and three — the process of introspection — we can examine our thoughts and feelings in order further to understand our own make-up. Indeed, this process of self-exploration seems to be essential if we are to be able to offer another person sustained attention.

If we constantly bottle-up problems we will find ourselves distracted by what the client has to say. Typically, when they begin to talk of a problem of theirs that is also a problem for us, we will suddenly find our attention distracted to zone two. Suddenly we will find ourselves pondering on our own problems and not those of the client. Regular self-examination can help us to clear away, at least temporarily, some of the more pressing personal problems that we experience. A case, perhaps, of 'counsellor, counsel thyself'!

Such exploration can be carried out either in isolation, in pairs or in groups. The skills exercises section of this book offers practical suggestions as to how such exploration can be developed. If performed in isolation, meditative techniques can be of value. Often, however, the preference will be to conduct such exploration in pairs or groups. In this way, we gain further insight through hearing other people's thoughts, feelings and observations and we can make useful comparisons between other people's experience and our own.

There are a variety of formats for running self-awareness groups, including sensitivity groups, encounter groups, groups therapy and training groups. Such groups are often organized by colleges and extra-mural departments of universities but they can also be set up on a 'do-it-yourself' basis. Ernst and Goodison (1981) offer some particularly useful guidelines for setting up, running and maintaining a self-help group for self-exploration.

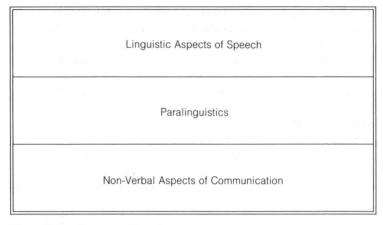

Figure 4.2. Aspects of listening

Such a group is useful as a means of developing self-awareness, as a peer support group for talking through counselling problems and also as a means of developing further counselling skills. Trying out new skills in a safe and trusting environment is often a better proposition than trying them out with real clients!

LISTENING

Listening is the process of 'hearing' the other person. This involves not only noting the things that they say, but also a whole range of other aspects of communication. Figure 4.2 outlines some of the things that can be noted during listening. Given the wide range of ways in which one person tries to communicate with another, this is further evidence of the need to develop the ability to offer close and sustained attention, as outlined above. Three aspects of listening are noted in the diagram. Linguistic aspects of speech refer to the actual words that the client uses, to the phrases they choose and to the metaphors they use to convey how they are feeling. Attention to such metaphors is often useful as metaphorical language can often convey more than can more conventional use of language (Cox, 1978).

Paralinguistics refer to all those aspects of speech that are not words. Thus, timing, volume, pitch and accent are all paralinguistic aspects of communication. They can offer us indicators of how the other person is feeling beyond the words that they use. Again, however, we must be careful of making assumptions and slipping into zone three, the zone of fantasy. Paralinguistics can only offer us a possible clue to how the other person is feeling. It is important that we check with the client the degree to which that clue matches with the client's own perception of the way they feel.

Non-verbal aspects of communication refer to 'body language': the way that the client expressed himself through the use of his body. Thus facial expression, use of gestures, body position and movement, proximity to the health care professional, touch in relation to the counsellor, all offer further clues about the client's internal status beyond the words they use and can be 'listened' to by the attentive health care professional. Again, any assumptions that we make about what such body language means need to be clarified with the client.

There is a temptation to believe that body language can be 'read', as if we all used it in the same sort of way. This is, perhaps, encouraged by works such as Desmond Morris's (1978) *Manwatching*. Reflection on the subject, however, will reveal that body language is dependent to a large degree on a wide number of variables: the context in which it occurs, the nature of the relationship, the individual's personal style and preference, the personality of the person 'using' the body language, and so on. It is safer, therefore, not to assume that we know what another person is 'saying' with their body language but, again, to treat it as a clue and to clarify with the client what he means. Thus it is preferable in counselling merely to bring to the client's attention the way they are sitting, or their facial expression, rather than offer an interpretation of it. Two examples may help here. In the first, the health care professional is offering an interpretation and an assumption:

I notice from the way that you have your arms folded and from your frown that you are uncomfortable with discussing things at home.

In the second example, the health care professional merely feeds back to the client what she observes and allows the client to clarify his situation:

I notice that you have your arms folded and that you're frowning. What are you feeling at the moment?

LEVELS OF LISTENING

The skilled health care professional learns to listen to all three aspects of communication and tries to resist the temptation to interpret what she hears. Three levels of listening may be identified:

Linguistic Aspects
Words,
Phrases,
Metaphors,
etc.

Paralinguistic Aspects:
Timing,
Volume,
Pitch,
Accent,
'Ums and errs,'
Fluency,
etc.

Non-Verbal Aspects of Communication
Facial expression,
Use of gesture,
Touch,
Body position,
Proximity to the health care professional,
Body movement,
Eye contact,
etc.

The first level of listening refers to the idea of the health care professional merely noting what is being said. In this mode, neither client nor health care professional are psychologically very 'close' and arguably the relationship will not develop very much. In the second level of listening, the health care professional learns to develop 'free floating' attention, i.e. she listens 'overall' to what is being said, as opposed to trying to catch every word.

Free floating attention also refers to 'going with' the client, of not trying to keep the client to a particular theme but of following the client's conversation wherever it goes. She also 'listens' to the client's non-verbal and paralinguistic behaviour as indicators of what the client is thinking and feeling. Faced with this deeper level of listening, the client feels a greater amount of empathy being offered by the health care professional. The health care professional begins to enter the frame of reference of the client and to explore his perceptual world. She begins to see the world as the client experiences it.

In the third level of listening, the health care professional maintains free floating attention, notices non-verbal and paralinguistic aspects of communication but also notices her own internal thoughts, feelings and body sensations. As Rollo May (1983) notes, it is frequently the case that what the health care professional is feeling, once the counselling relationship has deepened, is a direct mirror image of what the client is feeling. Thus the health care professional sensitively notices changes in herself and gently checks these with the client. It is as though the health care professional is listening both to the client and to herself and carefully using herself as a sounding board for how the relationship is developing. Watkins (1978) has described this process as 'resonance' and points out that this process is different from that of empathizing.

Rogers says that empathy means understanding the feelings of another. He holds that the therapist does not necessarily himself experience the feelings. If he did, that would be identification, and this is not the same as empathy. Resonance is a type of identification which is temporary (Watkins, 1978).

The use of the process of resonance needs to be judged carefully. Whilst it does not involve interpreting or offering a theory about what the client is feeling, it does offer a particularly close form of listening which can make the client feel listened to and fully understood. It is notable, too, that in these circumstances the client will often feel more comfortable with periods of silence as he struggles to verbalize his thoughts and feelings. Arguably, he allows these silences because he senses that the health care professional is 'with him' more completely than at other levels of listening. The net result of this deeper level of listening is that a truly empathic relationship develops. The client feels listened to, the health care professional feels she is understanding the client and a level of mutuality is achieved in which both people are communicating, both rationally and intuitively.

USE OF 'MINIMAL PROMPTS'

Whilst the health care professional is listening to the client, it is important that she shows that she is listening. An obvious aid to this is the use of what may be described as 'minimal prompts' — the use of head nods, 'yes's', 'mm's' and so on. All of these indicate that 'I am with you'. On the other hand, overuse of them can be irritating to the client, particularly, perhaps, the thoughtless and repetitive nodding of the head — the 'dog in the back of the car' phenomenon! It is important that the health care professional, at least initially, is consciously aware of her use of minimal prompts and tries to vary her repertoire. It is important also to note that very often such prompts are not necessary at all. Often, all the client needs is to be listened to and appreciates that the health care professional is listening, without the need for further reinforcement of the fact.

BEHAVIOURAL ASPECTS OF LISTENING

One other consideration to needs be made regarding the process of listening and that is the behaviours the health care professional adopts when listening to the client. Egan (1990) offers the acronym S.O.L.E.R. as a means of identifying and remembering the sorts of counsellor behaviour that encourage effective listening. The acronym is used as follows:

Sit squarely in relation to the client,
maintain an Open position,
Lean slightly towards the client,
maintain reasonable Eye contact with the client,
Relax!

First, the health care professional is encouraged to sit squarely in relation to the client. This can be understood both literally and metaphorically. In North America and the UK it is generally acknowledged that one person listens to another more effectively if she sits opposite or nearly opposite the other person, rather than next to him. Sitting opposite allows the health care professional to see all aspects of communication, both paralinguistic and non-verbal, that might be missed if she sat next to the client.

Second, the health care professional should consider adopting an open position in relation to the client. Again, this can be understood both literally and metaphorically. A 'closed' attitude is as much a block to effective counselling as is a closed body position. Crossed arms and legs, however, can convey a defensive feeling to the client and counselling is often more effective if the health care professional sits without crossing either. Having said that, many people feel more comfortable sitting with their legs crossed, so perhaps some licence should be used here. What should be avoided is the position where the health care professional sits in a 'knotted' position with both arms and legs crossed.

It is helpful if the health care professional appreciates that they can lean towards the client. This can encourage the client and make them feel more understood. If this does not seem immediately clear, next time you talk to someone, try leaning away from the other person and note the result.

Eye contact with the client should be reasonably sustained and a good rule of thumb is that the amount of eye contact that the health care professional uses should roughly match the amount the client uses. It is important, however, that the health care professional's eyes should be available for the client: the health care professional is always prepared to maintain eye contact. On the other hand it is important that the client does not feel stared at, nor intimidated by the health care professional's glare. Conscious use of eye contact can ensure that the client feels listened to and understood but not uncomfortable.

The amount of eye contact the health care professional can make will depend on a number of factors, including the topic under discussion, the degree of 'comfortableness' the health care professional feels with the client, the degree to which the health care professional feels attracted to the client, the amount of eye contact the client makes, the nature and quality of the client's eye contact, etc. If the health care professional continually finds the maintenance of eye contact difficult it is perhaps useful to consider talking the issue over with a trusted colleague or with a peer support group, for eye contact is a vital channel of communication in most interpersonal encounters (Heron, 1970).

Finally, it is important that the health care professional feels relaxed while listening. This usually means that she should refrain from 'rehearsing responses' in her head. It means that she gives herself up completely to the task of listening and trusts herself that she will make an appropriate response when she has to. This underlines the need to consider listening as the most important aspect of counselling. Everything else is secondary to it.

Many people feel that they have to have a ready response when engaged in a conversation with another person. In counselling, however, the main focus of the conversation is the client. The health care professional's verbal responses, although important, must be secondary to what the client has to say. Thus all the health care professional has to do is to sit back and listen intently. Easily said but not so easily done! The temptation to 'overtalk' is often great but can lessen with more experience and by making a conscious decision not to make too many verbal interventions.

All of these behavioural considerations can help the listening process. In order to be effective, however, they need to be used consciously. The health care professional needs to pay attention to using them and choose to use them. As we have noted, at first this conscious use of self will feel uncomfortable and unnatural. Practice makes it easier and with that practice comes the development of the health care professional's own style of working and behaving in the counselling relationship. No such style can develop if, first, the health care professional does not consciously consider the way she sits and the way she listens.

In summary, it is possible to identify some of those things which act as blocks to effective listening and some aids to effective listening. No doubt the reader can add to both these lists and such additions will be useful in that they will be a reflection of your own strengths and limitations as a listener.

Blocks to effective listening

- the health care professional's own problems
- health care professional's stress and anxiety
- awkward/uncomfortable seating
- lack of attention to listening behaviour
- value-judgements and interpretations on the part of the health care professional — health care professional's attention focused 'in' rather than 'out'
- 'rehearsals' inside the health care professional's head

Aids to effective listening

- attention focused 'out'
- suspension of judgement by the health care professional

- attention to the behavioural aspects of listening
- comfortable seating
- avoidance of interpretation
- judicious use of minimal prompts

SUMMARY OF THIS CHAPTER

The skills of attending and listening are essential ones that can be used in every health professional's job. The skills are clearly not limited only to use within a counselling relationship but can be applied in other interpersonal exchanges. An advantage of paying attention to the development of these particular skills is that becoming an effective listener not only makes for better practice but interpersonal effectiveness and self-awareness are also enhanced.

REFERENCES

Cox, M. (1978) *Structuring the Therapeutic Process*, Pergamon, London.
Egan, G. (1990) *The Skilled Helper*, 4th edn, Brooks/Cole, Pacific Grove, California.
Epting, F. (1984) *Personal Construct Counselling and Psychotherapy*, Wiley, Chichester.
Ernst, S. and Goodison, C. (1981) *In Your Own Hands: A Book of Self-Help Therapy*, Womens Press, London.
Heron, J. (1970) *The Phenomenology of the Gaze*, Human Potential Research Centre, University of Surrey, Guildford, Surrey.
May, R. (1983) Answer to Ken Wilber and John Rowan, *Journal of Humanistic Psychology*, **29**, vol. 2, 244–8.
Morris, D. (1978) *Manwatching*, Triad/Panther, St Albans.
Watkins, J. (1978) *The Therapeutic Self*, Human Sciences Press, New York.

5

Counselling skills

Aims of the chapter

The following issues and skills are discussed in this chapter:

- what is counselling?
- counselling skills
- coping with emotional release

WHAT IS COUNSELLING?

Counselling is the process of sitting and talking to a client, patient or colleague with the intention of helping them to arrive at decisions about how to act. The action element of counselling comes after the counselling session. In a sense, the counsellor rarely sees the outcome of his or her work. The counselling session may be the place where things are talked about: the *action* takes place away from that session, in the person's every-day life. The client-centred approach to counselling is perhaps the one most widely used today in the caring and health professions and is the one discussed here. It is notable, however, that other, equally effective methods exist, notably the cognitive approach and the more directive and prescriptive approaches described elsewhere (Burnard, 1989).

COUNSELLING SKILLS

Counselling skills may be divided into two sub-groups: a) listening and attending and b) counselling interventions. Listening and attending were considered in the last chapter. This chapter identifies important counselling interventions — the things that the health care professional says in the counselling relationship.

The term 'client-centred', first used by Carl Rogers (1951), refers to the notion that it is the client himself who is best able to decide how to find the solutions to their problems in living. 'Client-centred' in this sense may be contrasted with the idea of 'counsellor-centred' or 'professional-centred', both of which may suggest that someone other than the client is the 'expert'. Whilst this may be true when applied to certain concrete 'factual' problems — housing, surgery, legal problems, etc. — it is difficult to see how it can apply to personal life issues. In such cases, it is the client who identifies the problem and the client who, given time and space, can find his way through the problem to the solution.

Murgatroyd (1985) summarizes the client-centred position as:

- a person in need has come to you for help,
- in order to be helped they need to know that you have understood how they think and feel,
- they also need to know that, whatever your own feelings about who or what they are or about what they have or have not done, you accept them as they are,
- you accept their right to decide their own lives for themselves,
- in the light of this knowledge about your acceptance and understanding of them they will begin to open themselves to the possibility of change and development,
- but if they feel that their association with you is conditional upon them changing, they may feel pressurised and reject your help.

The first issue identified by Murgatroyd is the fact of the client coming for help and needing to be understood and accepted. What we need to consider now are ways of helping the person to express themselves, to open themselves and thus to begin to change. It is worth noting, too, the almost paradoxical nature of Murgatroyd's last point: that if the client feels that their association with you is conditional upon them changing, they may reject your help. Thus we enter into the counselling relationship without even being desirous of the other person changing.

In a sense, this is an impossible state of affairs. If we did not hope for change, we presumably would not enter into the task of counselling in the first place. On another level, however, the point is a very important one. People change at their own rate and in their own time. The process cannot be rushed and we cannot will another person to change. Nor can we expect them to change to become more the sort of person that we would like them to be. We must meet them on their own terms and observe change as they wish and will it to be (or not, as the case may be). This sort of counselling, then, is very altruistic. It demands of us that we make no demands of others.

Client-centred counselling is a process rather than a particular set of skills. It evolves through the relationship that the health care professional has with the client and vice versa. In a sense, it is a period of growth for both parties, for each learns from the other. It also involves the exercise of restraint. The health care professional must restrain herself from offering advice and from the temptation to put the client's life right for him.

The outcome of such counselling cannot be predicted nor can concrete goals be set (unless they are devised by the client, at their request). In essence, client-centred counselling involves an act of faith — a belief in the other person's ability to find solutions through the process of therapeutic conversation and through the act of being engaged in a close relationship with another human being.

Certain basic client-centred skills may be identified, although, as we have noted, it is the total relationship that is important. Skills exercised in isolation amount to little: the warmth, genuineness and positive regard must also be present. On the other hand, if basic skills are not considered, then the counselling process will probably be shapeless or it will degenerate into the health care professional becoming prescriptive. The skill of standing back and allowing the client to find his own way is a difficult one to learn. The following skills may help in the process.

- questions
- reflection
- selective reflection
- empathy building
- checking for understanding

Each skill can be learned. In order for that to happen, each must be tried and practised. There is a temptation to say 'I do that anyway!' when reading a description of some of these skills. The point is to notice the doing of them and to practise doing them better. Whilst counselling often shares the characteristics of everyday conversation, if it is to progress beyond that it is important that some, if not all, of the following skills are used effectively, tactfully and skilfully.

QUESTIONS

Two main sorts of questions may be identified in the client-centred approach: closed and open questions. A closed question is one that elicits a 'yes', 'no' or similar one-word answer. Or it is one to which the health care professional can anticipate an approximation of the answer, as she asks it. Examples of closed questions are as follows:

- What is your name?
- How many children do you have?
- Are you happier now?
- Are you still depressed?

Too many closed questions can make the counselling relationship seem like an interrogation! They also inhibit the development of the client's telling of his story and place the locus of responsibility in the relationship firmly with the client. Consider, for instance, the following exchange between marriage guidance counsellor and client:

> Counsellor: 'Are you happier now . . . at home?'
> Client: 'Yes, I think I am . . .'
> Counsellor: 'Is that because you can talk more easily with your wife?'
> Client: 'I think so . . . we seem to get on better, generally.'
> Counsellor: 'And has your wife noticed the difference?'
> Client: 'Yes, she has.'

In this conversation, made up only of closed questions, the counsellor clearly leads the conversation. She also tends to try to influence the client towards accepting the idea that he is 'happier now' and that his wife has 'noticed the difference'. One of the problems with this sort of questioning is that it gives little opportunity for the client profoundly to disagree with the counsellor. In the above exchange, for example, could the client easily have disagreed with the counsellor? It would seem not.

On the other hand, the closed question is useful in clarifying certain specific issues. For example, one may be used as follows:

> Client: 'It's not always easy at home . . . the children always seem to be so noisy . . . and my wife finds it difficult to cope with them . . .'
>
> Counsellor: 'How many children have you?'
>
> Client: 'Three. They're all under ten and they're at the sort of age when they use up a lot of energy and make a lot of noise . . .'

Here, the closed question is fairly unobtrusive and serves to clarify the conversation. Notice, too, that once the question has been asked, the counsellor allows the client to continue to talk about his family, without further interruption.

Open questions

Open questions are those that do not elicit a particular answer: the health care professional cannot easily anticipate what an answer will 'look like'. Examples of open questions include:

- What did you do then?
- How did you feel when that happened?
- How are you feeling right now?
- What do you think will happen?

Open questions are ones that encourage the client to say more, to expand on their story or to go deeper. An example of their use is as follows:

> Counsellor: 'What is happening at home at the moment?'
>
> Client: 'Things are going quite well. Everyone's much more settled now and my son's found himself a job. He's been out of work for a long time . . .'
>
> Counsellor: 'How have you felt about that?'
>
> Client: 'It's upset me a lot . . . It seemed wrong that I was

working and he wasn't . . . he had to struggle for a long time . . . he wasn't happy at all . . .'

Counsellor: 'And how are you feeling right now?'

Client: 'Upset . . . I'm still upset . . . I still feel that I didn't help him enough . . .'

In this conversation, the health care professional uses only open questions and the client expands on what he thinks and feels. More importantly, perhaps, the above example illustrates the health care professional 'following' the client and noting his paralinguistic and non-verbal cues. In this way, she is able to help the client to focus more on what is happening in the present.

Open questions are generally preferable, in counselling, to closed ones. They encourage longer, more expansive answers and are rather more free of value judgements and interpretation than are closed questions. All the same, the health care professional has to monitor the 'slope' of intervention when using open questions. It is easy, for example, to become intrusive by asking too piercing questions, too quickly. As with all counselling interventions, the timing of the use of questions is vital.

WHEN TO USE QUESTIONS

Questions can be used in the counselling relationships for a variety of purposes. The main ones include:

- Exploration: 'What else happened . . . ?', 'How did you feel then?'
- For Further Information: 'How many children have you got?', 'What sort of work were you doing before you retired?'
- To Clarify: 'I'm sorry, did you say you are to move or did you say you're not sure?', 'What did you say then . . . ?'
- Encouraging Client to Talk: 'Can you say more about that?', 'What are your feelings about that?'.

OTHER SORTS OF QUESTIONS

There are other ways of classifying questions and some to be avoided.

Leading questions

These are questions that contain an assumption which places the client in an untenable position. The classic example of a leading question is: 'Have you stopped beating your wife?' Clearly, however the question is answered, the client is in the wrong! Other examples of leading questions are:

> Is your depression the thing that's making your work so difficult? Are your family upset by your behaviour? Do you think that you may be hiding something — even from yourself?

The latter, pseudo-analytical questions are particularly awkward. What could the answer possibly be?

Value-laden questions

Questions such as 'Does your homosexuality make you feel guilty?', not only poses a moral question but guarantees that the client feels difficult answering it!

'Why' questions

These have been discussed in Chapter 3 and the problems caused by them in the counselling relationship suggest that they should be used very sparingly, if at all.

Confronting questions

Examples of these may include: 'Can you give me an example of when that happened?' and 'Do you still love your wife?'. Confrontation in counselling is quite appropriate once the relationship has fully developed but needs to be used skilfully and appropriately. It is easy for apparent 'confrontation' to degenerate into moralizing. Heron (1986) and Schulman (1982) offer useful approaches to effective confrontation in counselling.

FUNNELLING

Funnelling refers to the use of questions to guide the conversation from the general to the specific (Kahn and Cannel, 1957). Thus, the conversation starts with broad, open questions and slowly, more specific questions are used to focus the discussion. An example of the use of funnelling is as follows:

Counsellor: 'You seem upset at the moment, what's happening?'
Client: 'It's home . . . things aren't working out . . .'
Counsellor: 'What's happening at home?'
Client: 'I'm always falling out with Sarah and the children . . .'
Counsellor: 'What does Sarah feel about what's happening?'
Client: 'She's angry with me . . .'
Counsellor: 'About something in particular?'
Client: 'Yes, about the way I talk to Daren, my son . . .'
Counsellor: 'What is the problem with Daren?'

In this way, the conversation becomes directed and focused — and this may pose a problem. If the health care professional does use funnelling in this way, it is arguable that the counselling conversation is no longer client-centred but counsellor-directed. Perhaps, in many situations — particularly where shortage of time is an issue — a combination of following and leading may be appropriate. Following refers to the health care professional taking the lead from the client and exploring the avenues that he wants to explore. Leading refers to the health care professional taking a more active role and pursuing certain issues that she feels are important. If in doubt, however, the 'following' approach is probably preferable as it keeps the locus of control in the counselling relationship firmly with the client.

REFLECTION

Reflection (sometimes called 'echoing') is the process of reflecting back or paraphrasing the last few words that the client has used, in order to encourage them to say more. It is as though the health care professional is echoing the client's thoughts and as though that echo serves as a prompt. It is important that the reflection does not turn into a question and this is best achieved by the health care professional making the repetition in much the same tone of voice as the client used. An example of the use of reflection is as follows:

> Client: 'We had lived in the South for a number of years. Then we moved and I suppose that's when things started to go wrong . . .'
>
> Counsellor: 'Things started to go wrong . . .'
>
> Client: 'Well, we never really settled down. My wife missed her friends and I suppose I did really . . . though neither of us said anything.'
>
> Counsellor: 'Neither of you said that you missed your friends . . .'
>
> Client: 'We both tried to protect each other, really. I suppose if either of us had said anything, we would have felt that we were letting the other one down.'

In this example, the reflections are unobtrusive and unnoticed by the client. They serve to help the client to say more, to develop his story. Used skilfully and with good timing, reflection can be an important method of helping the client. On the other hand, if it is overused or used clumsily, it can appear stilted and is very noticeable. Unfortunately, it is an intervention that takes some practice and one that many people anticipate learning on counselling courses. As a result, when people return from counselling courses, their friends and relatives are often waiting for them to use the technique and may comment on it. This should not be a deterrent as the method remains a useful and therapeutic one.

SELECTIVE REFLECTION

Selective reflection refers to the method of repeating back to the client a part of something he said that was emphasized in some way or which seemed to be emotionally charged. Thus selective reflection draws from the middle of the client's utterance and not from the end. An example of the use of selective reflection is as follows:

> Client: 'We had just got married. I was very young and I thought things would work out O.K. We started buying our own house. My wife hated the place! It was important, though . . . we had to start somewhere . . .'

Counsellor: 'Your wife hated the house.'

Client: 'She thought it was the worst place she'd lived in! She reckoned that she would only live there for a year at the most and we ended up being there for five years!'

The use of selective reflection allowed the client in this example to develop further an almost throw-away remark. Often, these 'asides' are the substance of very important feelings and the health care professional can often help in the release of some of these feelings by using selective reflection to focus on them. Clearly concentration is important, in order to note the points on which to reflect selectively. Also, the counselling relationship is a flowing, evolving conversation which tends to be 'seamless'. Thus, it is little use the health care professional storing up a point which she feels would be useful to reflect selectively. By the time a break comes in the conversation, the item will probably be irrelevant!

This points up, again, the need to develop 'free floating attention': the ability to allow the ebb and flow of the conversation to go where the health care professional takes it and for the health care professional to trust her own ability to choose an appropriate intervention when a break occurs.

EMPATHY BUILDING

This refers to the health care professional making statements to the client that indicate that she has understood the feeling that the client is experiencing. A certain intuitive ability is needed here, for often empathy building statements refer more to what is implied than what is overtly said. An example of the use of empathy building statements is as follows:

Client: 'People at work are the same. They're all tied up with their own friends and families . . . they don't have a lot of time for me . . . though they're friendly enough . . .'

Health care professional: 'You sound angry with them . . .'

Client: 'I suppose I am! Why don't they take a bit of time to ask me how I'm getting on? It wouldn't take much! . . .'

Health care professional: 'It sounds as though you are saying that people haven't had time for you for a long time . . .'

Client: 'They haven't. My family didn't bother much . . . I

71

mean, they looked as though they did . . . but they didn't really . . .'

The empathy building statements used here are ones that read between the lines. Sometimes such reading between the lines can be completely wrong and the empathy building statement is rejected by the client. It is important when this happens for the health care professional to drop the approach altogether and to pay more attention to listening. Inaccurate empathy building statements often indicate an overwillingness on the part of the health care professional to become 'involved' with the client's perceptual world — at the expense of accurate empathy! Used skilfully, however, they help the client to disclose further and indicate to the client that they are understood.

CHECKING FOR UNDERSTANDING

Checking for understanding involves either a) asking the client if you have understood them correctly or b) occasionally summarizing the conversation in order to clarify what has been said. The first type of checking is useful when the client quickly covers a lot of topics and seems to be thinking aloud. It can be used to focus further the conversation or as a means of ensuring that the client really stays with what the client is saying. The second type of checking should be used sparingly or the counselling conversation can seem rather mechanical and studied. The following two examples illustrate the two uses of checking for understanding.

a)

  Client: 'I feel all over the place at the moment . . . things aren't quite right at work . . . money is still a problem and I don't seem to be talking to anyone . . . I'm not sure about work . . . sometimes I feel like packing it in . . . at other times I think I'm doing O.K . . .'
  Health care professional: 'Let me just clarify . . . you're saying things are generally a problem at the moment and you've thought about leaving work?'
  Client: 'Yes . . . I don't think I will stop work but if I can get to talk it over with my boss, I think I will feel easier about it.'

b)

> Health care professional: 'Let me see if I can jump sum up what we've talked about this afternoon. We talked over the financial problems and the question of talking to the bank manager. You suggested that you may ask him for a loan. Then you went on to say how you felt you could organize your finances better in the future . . . ?'
>
> Client: 'Yes, I think that covers most things . . .'

Some health care professionals prefer to use the second type of checking at the end of each counselling session and this may help to clarify things before the client leaves. On the other hand, there is much to be said for not 'tidying up' the end of the session in this way. If the loose ends are left, the client continues to think about all the issues that have been discussed as he walks away from the session. If everything is summarized too neatly, the client may feel that the problems can be 'closed down' for a while or, even worse, that they have been solved! Personal problems are rarely simple enough to be summarized in a few words and checking at the end of a session should be used sparingly.

These, then, are particular skills that encourage self-direction on the part of the client and can be learned and used by the health care professional. They form the basis of all good counselling and can always be returned to as a primary way of working with the client in the counselling relationship.

HELPING WITH EMOTIONS

A considerable part of the process of helping people in counselling is concerned with the emotional or 'feelings' side of the person. In the UK and North American cultures, a great premium is paced on the individual's being able to 'control' feelings and thus overt expression of emotion is often frowned upon. As a result, we learn to bottle-up feelings, sometimes from a very early age. In this chapter, we will consider the effects of such suppression of feelings and identify some practical ways of helping people to identify and explore their feelings. The skills involved in managing feelings can be seen to augment the skills discussed in the previous chapter — the basic client-centred counselling skills.

TYPES OF EMOTION

Heron (1977) distinguishes between at least four types of emotion, that are commonly suppressed or bottled-up: anger, fear, grief and embarrassment. He notes a relationship between these feelings and certain overt expressions of them. Thus, in counselling, anger may be expressed as loud sound, fear as trembling, grief through tears and embarrassment by laughter. He notes also a relationship between those feelings and certain basic human needs. Heron argues that we all have the need to understand and know what is happening to us. If that knowledge is not forthcoming, we may experience fear. We also need to make choices in our lives and, if those are restricted in certain ways, we may feel anger.

Thirdly, we need to experience the expression of love and of being loved. If that love is denied us or taken way from us, we may experience grief. To Heron's basic human needs may be added the need for self-respect and dignity. If such dignity is denied us, we may feel self-conscious and embarrassed. Practical examples of how these relationships 'work' in everyday life and in the counselling relationship may be illustrated as follows:

A 20-year-old girl is attempting to live in a flat on her own. Her parents, however, insist on visiting her regularly and making suggestions as to how she should decorate the flat. They also regularly buy her articles for it and gradually she senses that she is feeling very uncomfortable and distanced from her parents. In the counselling relationship she discovers that she is very angry: her desire to make choices for herself is continually being eroded by her parents' benevolence.

A 48-year-old man hears that his mother is seriously ill and, subsequently, she dies. He feels no emotions except that of feeling 'frozen' and unemotional. During a counselling session he suddenly discovers the need to cry profoundly. As he does so, he realizes that, many years ago, he had decided that crying was not a masculine thing to do. As a result, he blocked off his grief and felt numb, until, within the safety of the counselling relationship, he was able to discover his grief and express it.

A 17-year-old boy, discussing his college work, during a counselling session begins to laugh almost uncontrollably. As he does so, he begins to feel the laughter turning to tears.

Through his mixed laughter and tears he acknowledges that 'No-one ever took me seriously . . . not at school, at home . . . or anywhere'. His laughter may be an expression of his lack of self-esteem and his tears the grief he experiences at that lack.

In the last example it may be noted how emotions that are suppressed are rarely only of one sort. Very often, bottled-up emotion is a mixture of anger, fear, embarrassment and grief. Often, too, the causes of such blocked emotion are unclear and lost in the history of the person. What is perhaps more important is that the expression of pent-up emotion is often helpful in that it seems to allow the person to be clearer in his thinking once he has expressed it. It is as though the blocked emotion 'gets in the way' and its release acts as a means of helping the person to clarify his thoughts and feelings. It is notable that the suppression of feelings can lead to certain problems in living that may be clearly identified.

THE EFFECTS OF BOTTLING UP EMOTION

Physical discomfort and muscular pain

Wilhelm Reich, a psychoanalyst with a particular interest in the relationship between emotions and the musculature, noted that blocked emotions could become trapped in the body's muscle clusters (Reich, 1949). He noted that anger was frequently 'trapped' in the muscles of the shoulders, grief in muscles surrounding the stomach and fear in the leg muscles. Often, these trapped emotions lead to chronic postural problems. Sometimes, the thorough release of the blocked emotion can lead to a free of the muscles and an improved physical appearance. Reich believed in working directly on the muscle clusters in order to bring about emotional release and subsequent freedom from suppression and out of his work was developed a particular type of mind/body therapy, known as 'bioenergetics' (Lowen, 1967; Lowen and Lowen, 1977).

In terms of everyday counselling, trapped emotion is sometimes 'visible' in the way that the client holds himself and the skilled counsellor can learn to notice tension in the musculature and changes in breathing patterns that may suggest muscular tension. We have noted throughout this book how difficult it is to interpret another person's behaviour. What is important here is that such bodily manifestations are used only as a clue to what may be happening in the person. We cannot assume that a person who looks tense, is tense, until he has said that he is.

Health professionals will be very familiar with the link between body posture, the musculature and the emotional state of the person. Frequently, if patients and clients can be helped to relax, then their medical and psychological condition may improve more quickly. Those health professionals who deal most directly with the muscle clusters (remedial gymnasts and physiotherapists, for example) will tend to notice physical tension more readily but all carers can train themselves to observe these important indicators of the emotional status of the person in their care.

Difficulty in decision making

This is a frequent side-effect of bottled-up emotion. It is as though the emotion makes the person uneasy and that uneasiness leads to lack of confidence. As a result, that person finds it difficult to rely on his own resources and may find decision making difficult. When we are under stress of any sort it is often the case that we feel the need to check decisions with other people. Once some of this stress is removed, by talking through problems or by releasing pent-up emotions, the decision-making process often becomes easier.

Faulty self-image

When we bottle up feelings, those feelings often have an un-pleasant habit of turning against us. Thus, instead of express-ing anger towards others, we turn it against ourselves and feel depressed as a result, or, if we have hung onto unexpressed grief, we turn that grief in on ourselves and experience ourselves as less than we are. Often in counselling, as old resentments or dis-satisfactions are expressed, so the person begins to feel better about himself.

Setting unrealistic goals

Tension can lead to further tension. This tension can lead us to set ourselves unreachable targets. It is almost as though we set ourselves up to fail! Sometimes, too, failing is a way of punishing ourselves or it is 'safer' than achieving. Release of tension, through the expression of emotion, can sometimes help in a person taking a more realistic view of himself and his goal setting.

The development of long-term faulty beliefs

Sometimes, emotion that has been bottled-up for a long time can lead to a person's view of the world being coloured in a particular way. He learns that 'people can't be trusted' or 'people always let you down in the end'. It is as though old, painful feelings lead to distortions that become part of that person's world-view. Such long-term distorted beliefs about the world do not change easily but may be modified as the person comes to release feelings and learns to handle his emotions more effectively.

The 'last straw' syndrome

Sometimes, if emotion is bottled-up for a considerable amount of time, a valve blows and the person hits out — either literally or verbally. We have all experienced the problem of storing up anger and taking it out on someone else, a process that is sometimes called 'displacement'. The original object of our anger is now replaced by something or someone else. Again, talking through difficulties or the release of pent-up emotion can often help to ensure that the person does not feel the need to explode in this way.

Clearly, no two people react to the bottling-up of emotion in the same way. Some people, too, choose not to deal with life events emotionally. It would be curious to argue that there is a 'norm' where emotions are concerned. On the other hand, many people complain of being unable to cope with emotions and if the client perceives there to be a problem in the emotional domain, then that perception may be expressed as a desire to explore his emotional status.

It is important, however, that the counsellor does not force her particular set of beliefs about feelings and emotions on the client, but waits to be asked to help. Often the request for such help is a tacit request: the client talks about difficulty in dealing with emotion and that, in itself, may safely be taken as a request for help. A variety of methods is available to the counsellor to help in the exploration of the domain of feelings and those methods will be described. Sometimes, these methods produce catharsis: the expression of strong emotion — tears, anger, fear, laughter. Drawing on the literature on the subjects, the following statements may be made about the handling of such emotional release:

Emotional release is usually self-limiting. If the person is allowed to cry or get angry, that emotion will be expressed and then gradually subside. The supportive counsellor will allow it to happen and not become unduly distressed by it.

Physical support can sometimes be helpful in the form of holding the person's hand or putting an arm round them. Care should be taken, however, that such actions are unambiguous and that the holding of the client is not too 'tight'. A very tight embrace is likely to inhibit the release of emotion. It is worth remembering, also, that not everyone likes or wants physical contact. It is important that the counsellor's support is not seen as intrusive by the client.

Once the person has had a cathartic release they will need time to piece together the insights that they gain from such release. Often all that is needed is that the counsellor sits quietly with the client while he occasionally verbalizes what he is thinking. The post-cathartic period can be a very important stage in the counselling process.

There seems to be a link between the amount we can 'allow' another person to express emotion and the degree to which we can handle our own emotion. This is another reason why the counsellor needs self-awareness. To help others explore their feelings we need, first, to explore our own. Many colleges and university departments offer workshops on cathartic work and self-awareness development that can help in both training the counsellor to help others and in gaining self-insight.

Frequent 'cathartic counselling' can be exhausting for the counsellor and if she is to avoid 'burnout', she needs to set up a network of support from other colleagues or via a peer support group. We cannot hope constantly to handle other people's emotional release without its taking a toll on us.

METHODS OF HELPING THE CLIENT TO EXPLORE FEELINGS

These are practical methods that can be used in the counselling relationship to help the client to identify, examine and, if required, release emotion. Most of them will be more effective if the counsellor has first tried them on herself. This can be done simply by reading through the description of them and then trying them out in one's mind. Alternatively, they can be tried out with a colleague or friend. Another way of exploring their effectiveness is to use them in a peer support context. The setting up and running of such a group is described in the final chapter of this book, along with various exercises that can be used to improve counselling skills. All of the following activities should be used gently and thoughtfully and timed to fit in with the client's requirements. There should never be any sense of pushing the client to explore feelings because of a misplaced belief that 'a good cry will do him good!'

Giving permission

Sometimes in counselling, the client tries desperately to hang on to strong feelings and not to express them. As we have seen, this may be due to the cultural norm which suggests that holding on is often better than letting go. Thus a primary method for helping someone to explore his emotions is for the counsellor to 'give permission' for the expression of feeling. This can be done simply through acknowledging that 'It's alright with me if you feel you are going to cry . . . ' In this way the counsellor has reassured the client that expression of feelings is acceptable within the relationship. Clearly, a degree of tact is required here. It is important that the client does not feel pushed into expressing feelings that he would rather not express. The 'permission giving' should never be coercive nor should there be an implicit suggestion that 'you must express your feelings!'.

Literal description

This refers to inviting the client to go back in his memory to a place that he is, until now, only alluding to and describing that

79

place in some detail. An example of this use of literal description is as follows:

> Client: 'I used to get like this at home . . . I used to get very upset . . .'
> Counsellor: 'Just go back home for a moment . . . describe one of the rooms in the house . . .'
> Client: 'The front room faces directly out onto the street . . . there is an armchair by the window . . . the TV in the corner . . . our dog is lying on the rug . . . it's very quiet . . .'
> Counsellor: 'What are you feeling right now?'
> Client: 'Like I was then . . . angry . . . upset . . .'

The going back to a place that was the scene of an emotional experience and describing in literal terms can often bring that emotion back. When the counsellor has invited the client literally to describe a particular place, she then asks him to identify the feeling that emerges from that description. It is important that the description has an 'I am there' quality about it and does not slip into a detached description, such as: 'We lived in a big house which wasn't particularly modern but then my parents didn't like modern houses much . . .'

Locating and developing a feeling in terms of the body

As we have noted above, very often feelings are accompanied by a physical sensation. It is often helpful to identify that physical experience and to invite the client to exaggerate it, to allow the feeling to 'expand' in order to explore it further. Thus, an example of this approach is as follows:

> Counsellor: 'How are you feeling at the moment?'
> Client: 'Slightly anxious.'
> Counsellor: 'Where, in terms of your body, do you feel the anxiety?'
> Client: (rubs stomach): 'Here.'
> Counsellor: 'Can you increase that feeling in your stomach?'
> Client: 'Yes, its spreading up to my chest.'
> Counsellor: 'And what's happening now?'
> Client: 'It reminds me of a long time ago . . . when I first started work . . .'
> Counsellor: 'What happened there . . . ?'

Again, the original suggestion by the counsellor is followed through by a question to elicit how the client is feeling following the suggestion. This gives the client a chance to identify the thoughts that go with the feeling and to explore them further.

Empty chair

Another method of exploring feelings is to invite the client to imagine the feeling that they are experiencing as 'sitting' in a chair next to them and then have them address the feeling. This can be used in a variety of ways and the next examples show its applications:

a)

Client: 'I feel very confused at the moment, I can't seem to sort things out . . . '

Counsellor: 'Can you imagine your confusion sitting in that chair over there . . . what does it look like?'

Client: 'It looks like a great big ball of wool . . . how odd!'

Counsellor: 'If you could speak to your confusion, what would you say to it?'

Client: 'I wish I could sort you out!'

Counsellor: 'And what's your confusion saying back to you?'

Client: 'I'm glad you don't sort me out — I stop you from having to make any decisions!'

Counsellor: 'And what to you make of that?'

Client: 'I suppose that could be true . . . the longer I stay confused, the less I have to make decisions about my family . . . '

b)

Counsellor: 'How are you feeling about the people you work with . . . you said you found it quite difficult to get on with them . . . ?'

Client: 'Yes, it's still difficult, especially my boss.'

Counsellor: 'Imagine your boss is sitting in that chair over there . . . how does that feel?'

Client: 'Uncomfortable! He's angry with me!'

Counsellor: 'What would you like to say to him?'

Client: 'Why do I always feel scared of you . . . why do you make me feel uncomfortable?'

Counsellor: 'And what does he say?'
Client: 'I don't! It's you that feels uncomfortable, not me . . .
You make yourself uncomfortable . . . (to the counsellor)
He's right! I do make myself uncomfortable but I use him as
an excuse . . . '

The 'empty chair' can be used in a variety of ways to set up a
dialogue between either the client and his feelings or between
the client and a person that the client talks about. It offers a
very direct way of exploring relationships and feelings and deals
directly with the issue of 'projection' — the tendency we have to
see qualities in others that are, in fact, our own. Using the empty
chair technique can bring to light those projections and allow the
client to see them for what they are. Other applications of this
method are described in detail by Perls (1969).

Contradiction

It is sometimes helpful if the client is asked to contradict a
statement that they make, especially when that statement contains some ambiguity. An example of this approach is as follows:

Client: (looking at the floor): 'I've sorted everything out now:
everything's O.K.'
Counsellor: 'Try contradicting what you've just said . . .'
Client: 'Everything's not O.K. . . . Everything isn't sorted
out . . . (laughs) . . . that's true, of course . . . there's a lot
more to sort out yet . . .'

Mobilization of body energy

Developing the theme discussed above regarding the idea that
emotions can be trapped within the body's musculature, it is
sometimes helpful for the counsellor to suggest to the client that
he stretches, or takes some very deep breaths. In the process, the
client may become aware of tensions that are trapped in his body
and begin to recognize and identify those tensions. This, in turn,
can lead to the client talking about and expressing some of those
tensions. This is particularly helpful if, during the counselling
conversation, the client becomes less and less 'mobile' and adopts

a particularly hunched or curled-up position in his chair. The invitation to stretch serves almost as a contradiction to the body position being adopted by the client at that time.

Exploring fantasy

We often set fairly arbitrary limits on what we think we can and cannot do. When a client seems to be doing this, it is sometimes helpful to explore what may happen if this limit were broken. An example of this is as follows:

> Client: 'I'd like to be able to go abroad for a change, I never seem to go very far on holiday.'
> Counsellor: 'What stops you?'
> Client: 'Flying, I suppose . . .'
> Counsellor: 'What's the worst thing about flying?'
> Client: 'I get very anxious.'
> Counsellor: 'And what happens if you get very anxious?'
> Client: 'Nothing really! I just get anxious!'
> Counsellor: 'So nothing terrible can happen if you allow yourself to get anxious?'
> Client: 'No, not really . . . I hadn't thought about it like that before . . .'

Rehearsal

Sometimes the anticipation of a coming event or situation is anxiety provoking. The counsellor can usefully help the client to explore a range of feelings by rehearsing with him a future event. Thus the client who is anticipating a forthcoming interview may be helped by having the counsellor act the role of an interviewer, with a discussion afterwards. The client who wants to develop the assertive behaviour to enable him to challenge his boss may benefit from role playing the situation in the counselling session. In each case, it is important that both client and counsellor 'get into role' and that the session does not just become a discussion of what may or may not happen. The actual playing through and rehearsal of a situation is nearly always more powerful than a discussion of it.

Alberti and Emmons (1982) offer some useful suggestions

about how to set up role plays and exercises for developing assertive behaviour and Wilkinson and Canter (1982) describe some useful approaches to developing socially skilled behaviour. Often, if the client can practise effective behaviour, then the appropriate thoughts and feelings can accompany that behaviour. The novelist, Kurt Vonnegut, wryly commented that: 'We are what we pretend to be — so take care what you pretend to be' (Vonnegut, 1969). Sometimes, the first stage in changing is trying out a new pattern of behaviour or a new way of thinking and feeling. Practice, therefore, is invaluable.

This approach develops from the idea that what we think influences what we feel and do. If our thinking is restrictive, we may begin to feel that we can or cannot do certain things. Sometimes if these barriers to feeling and doing are challenged a person may be freed to think, feel and act differently.

These methods of exploring feelings can be used alongside the client-centred interventions described in the previous chapter. They need to be practised in order that the counsellor feels confident in using them and the means to developing the skills involved are identified in the final chapter of this book. The domain of feelings is one that is frequently addressed in counselling. Counselling people who want to explore feelings takes time and cannot be rushed. Also, the development and use of the various skills described here is not the whole of the issue. Health professionals working with emotions need also to have developed the personal qualities that have been described elsewhere: warmth, genuineness, empathic understanding and unconditional positive regard. Emotional counselling can never be a mechanical process but is one that touches the lives of both client and counsellor.

SUMMARY OF THE CHAPTER

Counselling skills are the basic prerequisite for any effective health care professional. The skills discussed in this chapter are applicable in a wide range of health care settings.

REFERENCES

Alberti, R.E. and Emmons, M.L. (1982) *Your Perfect Right: a guide to assertive living*, Impact, San Luis Obispo, California.

Burnard, P. (1989) *Counselling Skills for Health Professionals*, Chapman and Hall, London.

Heron, J. (1977) *Catharsis in Human Development*, Human Potential Research Project, University of Surrey, Guildford, Surrey.

Heron, J. (1986) *Six Category Intervention Analysis*, 2nd edn, Human Potential Research Project, University of Surrey, Guildford, Surrey.

Kahn, R.L. and Cannel, C.F. (1957) *The Dynamics of Interviewing*, Wiley, New York.

Lowen, A. (1967) *Betrayal of the Body*, Macmillan, New York.

Lowen, A. and Lowen, L. (1977) *The Way to Vibrant Health: A manual of bioenergetic exercises*, Harper and Row, New York.

Murgatroyd, S. (1985) *Counselling and Helping*, Methuen, London.

Perls, F. (1969) *Gestalt Therapy Verbatim*, Real People Press, Lafayette, California.

Reich, W. (1949) *Character Analysis*, Simon and Schuster, New York.

Rogers, C.R. (1951) *Client-Centred Therapy*, Constable, London.

Schulman, E.D. (1982) *Intervention in the Human Services: a guide to skills and knowledge*, 3rd edn, Mosby, St Louis, Missouri.

Vonnegut, K. (1969) *Mother Night*, Gollancz, London.

Wilkinson, J. and Canter, S. (1982) *Social Skills Training Manual: Assessment, programme design and management of training*, Wiley, Chichester.

6

Group facilitation skills

Aims of the chapter

The following issues and skills are discussed in this chapter:

- types of groups
- group life
- group dynamics
- group facilitation skills

Health care professionals often need to facilitate groups. To run groups effectively and therapeutically, they have to make certain decisions about *how* they will run groups. This article considers aspects of group facilitation.

First, what sorts of groups are health care professionals likely to find themselves facilitating? A short list would include the following:

- education groups
- discussion groups
- therapy groups
- relative support groups
- case conferences
- curriculum planning groups
- stress/relaxation groups

Whilst each of these groups has different aims, the skills required to facilitate them are similar. The overall objective will be to enable a group of people to make the best possible use of the time that they have at their disposal. The health care professional acting as facilitator needs to notice her own style of facilitation and its strengths and deficits. Once those strengths and deficits have become explicit, the strengths can be reinforced and the deficits made good.

A MAP OF THE GROUP PROCESS

Tuckman (1965) offered a useful map of the group process. He noted that every group passes through four stages in its development and life. He described these as the stages of a) forming, b) storming, c) norming and d) performing. During stage one, the forming stage, group members meet each other for the first time and attempt to discover what behaviour is and is not required of them. This is a time for testing the water, of discovering other people and for discovering one's role in the group. In many ways, the new member of the group is 'on her best behaviour': the real person has yet to emerge.

In the storming stage, group members begin to thaw out a little. As a result they characteristically become hostile with one another as they battle to assert themselves and to stamp their personalities on the group. This is the stage of conflict between 'my' needs and wants and those of the group. Often this is a painful period in which there are fights for leadership of the group and attempts at establishing a pecking order. Health care professionals in the early stages of their education and training, for example, may notice the advent of the storming stage developing once the introductory period in the school or college has been worked through or towards the middle or end of their first year. In this stage, friendships and loyalties are tested and it may be a time when certain individuals either opt out of the group and leave the education and training course or feel pressurized to leave by the group.

Out of the storming stage develops the 'norming' stage, when the group comes to terms with itself and the individuals in it resolve their conflicts to some degree — both personal and interpersonal. In order for the group to function harmoniously, rules, both written and unwritten, are established in the group's resolve to become more cohesive. Members typically get to know one another better and a more trusting, intimate atmosphere develops. Health care professional education and training courses when they reach this stage are often perceived as having established themselves by their tutors or lecturers and fellow health care professionals. The group feels as though it has arrived!

The danger, here, is that such groups will become *too* settled and too complacent. There is also a problem when groups are too readily socialized into the norms of the institution. In this case, they tend to be readily accepting what they see and lose a certain critical faculty. It is important that all health care professionals maintain the ability to think critically and are able to challenge the prevailing practices in the clinical areas in which they work. In most large institutions there develops what has been called an 'organizational culture'. That is to say that institutions, as large groups themselves, develop their own norms and seek to initiate newcomers into those norms in order for things to go along much as they have in the past. The new health profession group not only has to develop its own norms but may find itself in conflict or disagreement with the norms of the organizational culture.

The norming stage leads on to the most productive phase of group life: the performing stage. Here, the group has developed a mature collective identity and its members are able to work easily and usefully together. The danger arises, again, in this stage that the group can become complacent and that new growth is not encouraged.

This can be seen in certain clinical environments where everyone has worked together for a considerable period and have come to know each other, their habits and behaviours, well. Such a group can become inward looking and reject both new ideas and new members. Students arriving in such groups often feel left out or feel that they are intruding. The group that arrives at the performing stage needs to keep itself alert to changes and suggestions from outside of itself.

'Groupthink', the term that is sometimes used to describe the tendency for groups to work as if they were one, closed-minded individual, can occur if the group does not remain in touch and awake to other groups and to new ideas. It could be argued that many health professional groups and perhaps the profession itself has a tendency towards such closed thinking.

This then is a typical cycle through which most groups seem to pass. It may be viewed as a life cycle of the group and is directly comparable to the life cycle of the individual: it mimics childhood, adolescence, young adulthood and maturity. Thus the life cycle of life as experienced by the individual is played out in the larger arena of the group. Viewed in this light, group experiences can be valuable for developing further individual awareness. The person who monitors her behaviour and responses in the group can gain insights into themselves through appreciating this correlation between the life cycle of the group and the life cycle of the individual.

The health care professional in the group may see herself as 'reliving' stages of her own life when she joins that group. The group is perhaps the most potent medium through which to develop self-awareness. In the group both self-disclosure and feedback from others are present — two vital ingredients for awareness.

If the metaphor of the life cycle of the group is accepted, it will be understood that a group may well reach the point where it has fulfilled its function and the group is disbanded. The cycle has been completed. In health care professional education and training this ending of the group life comes naturally at the end of a three- or four-year period because the life period for the group has been predetermined by the college, school or examining body. In other groups, however, such a time period may not be so clear cut and it is important that at intervals through any 'performing' period, the group reviews its performance and function. There is little value in continuing the group's existence when the point of its existence has been exhausted. There is nothing worse than belonging to a 'dead' group.

Second to the issue of the group's stages comes the question of the processes that occur during the group's life. All that happens in a group may be divided into a) content and b) processes. Content refers to all that is said and talked about in any given group. Processes are all those things that happen in a group — the dynamics of the group. Such processes occur in groups of all types. They are more noticeable in small, intimate groups but also frequently occur in professional and work groups. They have been so frequently noted that they are easily described.

Recognition of such processes is vital for anyone running groups and it is helpful if group members learn to recognize them; once again, developing such awareness is part of the larger task of developing personal awareness. It is often useful if the group facilitator holds a discussion about group processes at one of the early meetings of that group. She may also like to invite group members to notice these processes as they occur, thus a sense of group reflexivity occurs. Time can then be put aside at regular intervals to discuss the perceived processes. In self-awareness groups, discussion of processes are just as important as the discussion of content. It is regrettable that traditional educational methods have mostly concentrated on the content of courses and study periods at the expense of exploring processes.

GROUP PROCESSES

Typical group processes may thus be described. Pairing can be noted when two individuals, usually sitting next to each other, engage in a quiet and often hesitant conversation with each other. The conversation may occur as a series of 'asides', facial expression and, in the extreme form, in the passing of notes! Pairing is distracting for other group members and may occur as a result of disaffection with the group, insecurity on the part of one or both of the pair involved, boredom or as a means of testing group leadership. Another form of pairing can be seen when two group members form a fairly exclusive relationship and support each other in a determined manner whenever either of them makes a contribution to group affairs and particularly when either of them is under attack from any other group member.

Projection occurs when an individual identifies the group as being responsible for her feelings. The person sees a quality in the group which is, in fact, a quality of her own but of which she is unaware. Thus the individual may say 'this group is hostile and unfriendly', when it is plain to the rest of the group that such a description fits the group member herself. Such projection may arise out of insecurity in the group or out of the individual's own lack of awareness.

The process of 'owning' projections and taking responsibility for oneself can be a particularly valuable piece of experiential learning in the group. On the other hand, you have to be careful. Not everything that a person says about a group is a projection. Sometimes they are merely describing what is obviously true about the group. So how do you distinguish between a projection and a description? No easy task! Some guidelines that may help here are these:

a) a projection is usually only experienced by one person;
b) the rest of the group usually disagrees with a projection;
c) often the individual comes to recognize her own projections
   — especially if she is on the lookout for them;

d) descriptions are usually corroborated by other group members;

e) descriptions do not usually have the 'emotional tone' that can accompany projections.

Scapegoating often occurs during the 'storming' stage of the group. The group looks for someone to blame for the way they are feeling and behaving and chooses a fairly quiet or vulnerable member on whom to vent their feelings. In this sense, scapegoating is a type of collective bullying. Alternatively, the group finds an outside scapegoat and blames 'the organization' or 'the profession' for the circumstances in which it finds itself. This is the 'group beef'. Usually this blaming of outside organizations or bodies is a means of the group avoiding responsibility for itself or a way of avoiding making decisions. Recognition of such scapegoating is part of the group leader's role and identification of it by the group itself can lead to a sense of growing cohesion and personal awareness. Again, though, a word of caution. Sometimes the organization or the profession *is* to blame! It is important to make the distinction.

When a group member becomes 'shut-down' (Heron, 1973), they cut themselves off from the rest of the group, often feeling swamped by it and emotionally fragile. This may be caused by the group member suddenly identifying with a painful experience that is being described by someone else. It may be a response to the general emotional tone of the group or it may be a rejection of the ideas that are being put forward in the group discussion. The skilled group facilitator recognizes such shutting down and helps the individual either to express her feelings or quietly to rejoin the group. There will be occasions, too, when the group member favours a short break from the group. Shutting down often occurs when a group member begins to face important emotional issues that have been previously buried.

The shut-down person is in crisis. She cannot face her feelings and she cannot verbalize how she feels. Working through such a phase must be handled tactfully and sensitively and the person should never be rushed or told that expressing her pent-up feelings would 'do her good'. Sometimes it would, sometimes it wouldn't. The point is that it is the *group member*'s place to decide whether or not now is a good time to work through the bottled-up feelings.

The person who 'rescues' may be a 'compulsive carer'. She

91

may find it easier to defend others from attack than to let those people fend for themselves and learn from the experience. Often rescuing others is a means of avoiding dealing with personal problems — to be seen as the person who always comes to another's aid can serve as a smokescreen for covering unresolved conflicts. It may be that many health care professionals are compulsive carers. Often it is easier to care for others than it is to care for ourselves. This is fine as far as it goes but constantly caring and rescuing others is a recipe for burnout and emotional exhaustion.

Part of the process of developing self-awareness includes our standing back and enabling others to learn through experience rather than rushing in and helping too quickly. Often the temptation is to protect others from that which we cannot take ourselves. We feel that 'if I can't take it, she can't', forgetting that the other person is a *different* person and blurring the distinction between 'me' and 'you'. As we gain awareness and resilience, we can allow others to live through their own life without being overprotected or denied the chance to develop their own coping skills.

This applies to a wide range of health care situations: the patient who learns to cope with their anxiety develops the ability to cope with it again; the person who is allowed to live through a certain amount of pain develops the ability to deal with pain. If we constantly 'rescue' we constantly deny people the ability to develop autonomy.

There are, of course, limits to this. The group facilitator has responsibilities towards the members of her group and some judgements have to be made about the degree of rescuing that *she* can make. As a general rule, she may want to 'rescue' members who are being scapegoated in the early days of the group's development. As the group progresses, she can slowly rescue less and less and allow individuals to fend for themselves more and more.

The group process known as flight can be demonstrated in various ways. The group which avoids difficult issues or decisions can be said to be taking flight. The individual group member who is constantly humorous and lighthearted may also be taking flight in humour. The member who always has a theoretical explanation for everything may often be taking flight from feelings. Yet another form of flight is keeping group discussion and meetings on a superficial level, thus deep and more disturbing issues are kept safely at a distance. Identifying and working through flight is a means of helping the group to grow. Self-disclosure occurs more readily when flight is avoided and group members are able to share each other's experiences on an adult-to-adult basis.

Again, this is not to say that all laughter is flight or that the group should always be deep and profound. It is merely to acknowledge that we all escape from facing ourselves, especially in the company of others.

In looking at group processes, it is worth noting that the energy level of any group will fluctuate from time to time just as an individual's energy level will have its peaks and troughs. Part of the development of group life involves living through the periods of low energy and taking advantage of the peaks. Again, the skilful leader and skilful group member will *notice* such fluctuations, take responsibility for them and make adjustments as necessary. When group energy does drop, the following courses of action, by the facilitator, may be appropriate:

a) sit it out and see what happens;
b) suggest a change of activity;
c) draw the group's attention to the drop in energy;
d) take a short break.

CHARACTERISTICS OF ALL GROUPS

Finally, small groups have things in common. Dorothy Stock Whittington (1987) offers a useful list of the characteristics of groups. The list is as follows:

1. Groups develop particular moods and atmospheres.
2. Shared themes can build up in groups.
3. Groups evolve norms and belief systems.
4. Groups vary in cohesiveness and in the permeability of their boundaries.
5. Groups develop and change their character over a period of time.
6. Persons occupy different positions in groups with respect to power, centrality and being liked and disliked.
7. Individuals in groups sometimes find one or two other persons who are especially important to them because they are

similar in some respect to significant persons in the individual's life or to significant aspects of the self.
8. Social comparison can take place in a group.
9. A group is an environment in which persons can observe what others do and say and then observe what happens next.
10. A group is an environment in which persons can receive feedback from others concerning their own behaviour or participation.

Arguably, these characteristics are true of most small groups, from clinical case conferences to learning groups and from therapy groups to discussion groups. Walker's list offers considerable material for discussion with both peers and students and may be a useful starting point for the teaching about groups and group dynamics.

DIMENSIONS OF FACILITATOR STYLE

Heron (1989) offers a six-fold model of facilitator styles. These six aspects of facilitation he calls dimensions. These are a different and revised set to that presented in Chapter 1 of this book. It seems to me that *both* versions have much to commend them and the two versions can be used in a wide range of therapeutic and educational contexts. The dimensions are as follows:

- the planning dimension
- the meaning dimension
- the confronting dimension
- the feeling dimension
- the structuring dimension
- the valuing dimension

The six dimensions of facilitator style may be used to make decisions about how *this* group is run at *this* time. Not all of the dimensions will be used in every group. Decisions about which dimension will be used during which group will depend on the type of group that is being run, the aims of that group, the personality of the facilitator and the needs of the participants.
The dimensions cover most aspects of the setting up and running of groups. What follows is an adapted version of Heron's model.

THE PLANNING DIMENSION

This dimension is concerned with the setting up of the group. Group members always need to know *why* they are in a particular group. Therefore the group facilitator needs to make certain decisions about how to identify the aims and objectives of the group. She has at least three options:

1. She can decide upon the aims and objectives herself, before setting up the group at all.
2. She can negotiate the aims and objectives with the group. In this case, she will decide on some of those aims and objectives. The group will decide on others.
3. She can encourage the group to set its own aims and objectives. In this case, all the facilitator does is to turn up on a certain day with a 'title' or name for the group. All further decisions about what the group is to achieve are made by the group.

The first example above illustrates the traditional learning group approach. The health care professional educator who uses this approach will have set aims and objectives for a particular lesson that she has planned in advance.

The second example illustrates the negotiated group approach. The health care professional working as a group therapist (for example) will meet the group for the first time and work with them to identify what that group can achieve in the time that they meet together.

The third example illustrates the fully client-centred or student-centred approach to working with groups. Here, the health care professional does not anticipate the needs or wants of the group at all. Instead, she allows the learning, therapy or discussion group to set its own agenda. Such an approach needs careful handling if it is not to degenerate into an aimless series of meetings.

Other aspects of the planning dimension include making decisions about the following issues:

- the number of group participants;
- whether or not particular 'rules' will apply to the group;
- whether or not group membership will remain the same throughout the life of the group (the closed group) or whether new members will be allowed to join (the open group).

Again, such planning decisions can be taken either unilaterally by the facilitator or via negotiation with the group.

THE MEANING DIMENSION

This aspect of group facilitation is concerned with what sense group members make of being in the group. As with the previous dimension, at least three options are open here:

1. The health care professional can offer explanations, theories or models to enable group members to make sense of what is happening. Thus a health care professional running a support group for bereaved relatives may offer a theoretical model of bereavement to enable those relatives to have a framework for understanding what is happening to them.
2. The health care professional may sometimes offer 'interpretations' of what is going on. At other times, she will listen to group members' perceptions of what is happening. This may frequently happen in an open discussion group or a case conference.
3. The facilitator offers no explanations or theories but encourages group members to verbalize their own ideas, thoughts and theories. This is the non-directive mode of working with meaning in a group.

THE CONFRONTING DIMENSION

When people work together, all sorts of conflicts can arise. Sometimes these conflicts are overt and show themselves in arguments and disagreements. Sometimes, a 'hidden agenda' is at work. Conflicts sit just beneath the surface of group life. Whilst they affect it in various ways, they cannot be worked with unless the group addresses them directly. The confronting dimension of facilitation is concerned with ways in which individual members and the group as a whole are challenged. The three ways of working in this dimension are as follows:

1. The health care professional can challenge the group or its members directly. Thus, she asks questions, makes sugges-

tions, offers interpretations of behaviour in the group. Her aim is to encourage the group and its members to confront what is happening at various levels.

2. The health care professional can facilitate an atmosphere in which people feel safe enough to challenge each other (and the facilitator). In help in this process, the following 'ground rules' for direct and clear communication can help:
   a) Say 'I' rather than 'you', 'we' or 'people' when discussing issues in the group,
   b) Speak directly to other people, rather than about them. Thus 'I am angry with you, David' is better than 'I am angry with people in this group'.
3. The health care professional can choose not to confront at all. In this case, two things may happen:
   a) no confrontation takes place and the group gets 'stuck', or
   b) the group learns to challenge itself, without assistance from the facilitator.

The first example of confrontation above is the traditional 'chairperson' mode of facilitation. The health care professional who uses this approach stays in control of the group. The negotiated style of confrontation is one that can be used in discussion groups and informal teaching sessions. The third example is one that can be used in meetings and discussions that are of a very formal kind. If it is used in therapy and self-awareness groups, the chances are that the 'hidden agenda' will not be addressed or that the group members will outgrow the need for the facilitator. It is arguable that *all* groups should aim at becoming independent of the group leader.

THE FEELING DIMENSION

Therapy groups, self-awareness groups and certain sorts of learning groups tend to generate emotion in participants. The feeling dimension is concerned with how such emotional expression is dealt with. Decisions that can be made in this domain include the following:

1. Will emotional release be *encouraged*? This may be appropriate in a therapy or social skills training group.

GROUP FACILITATION SKILLS

2. Is there to be an explicit *contract* with the group about emotional release? Here, the health care professional may suggest
   at the beginning of the first group meeting that emotional
   release is 'allowed', thus giving group members permission to
   express emotions.
3. Does the health care professional feel skilled in handling emotional release? If not, she may want to develop skills in coping
   with other people's feelings, especially when these involve the
   overt expression of tears, anger or fear. Training in cathartic
   work is needed here.

THE STRUCTURING DIMENSION

Structure is a necessary part of group life. Without it, the group
can fall apart. The issue here is *how* such structure is developed.
Again, at least three options open up in this domain.

1. The health care professional can decide on the total structure
   of the group. In a social skills group, for example, she may
   introduce a variety of exercises and activities that allow participants to learn how to answer the telephone, introduce
   themselves at parties or take faulty goods back to a shop. At
   all times, she remains in control of the overall structure.
2. The health care professional can encourage group members to
   organize certain aspects of the life and structure of the group.
   Thus the ward sister who is running a learning group may
   invite students to read and discuss seminar papers. In this
   respect, she is handing over some of the structure to group
   members.
3. The health care professional can play a minimal role in structuring the life of the group. The extreme example of this is the
   'Tavistock' approach to group therapy in which the group
   starts and finishes at particular times. Between those times the
   facilitator makes no attempt to 'lead' the group. This is not for
   the uninitiated!

As a general rule it is probably better for the new facilitator to
start with lots of structure (which is imposed by her). As she
gains confidence in running groups, she can gradually hand over
some of that structure to group members.

THE VALUING DIMENSION

This aspect of group facilitation is concerned with creating a supportive and valuing atmosphere in which the group can work. No group will succeed if the atmosphere is one of distrust and suspicion. The issues here are the following:

1. Is the facilitator confident enough to allow disagreement, discussion and varieties of points of view?
2. Dose she have sufficient self-awareness to know the effect that she is having on the group?
3. Is she skilled, positive, life asserting and encouraging?

Learning to value other people (and oneself) comes with experience of running groups, developing a range of therapeutic skills such us counselling, social skills and assertiveness.

Facilitation can be an exhilarating and educational experience for health care professionals and educators. The skills involved have wide application within the field of health care. Used effectively, such skills can have direct and indirect effects on improving the quality of education, management and care. This chapter has described some of the sorts of decisions that the new facilitator may want to make about how to run clinical, managerial or training groups.

SUMMARY OF THE CHAPTER

This chapter has identified the specific skills of working in group settings. Most health care professionals need to become proficient in working with people in groups. The skills identified here have broad application across the professions.

REFERENCES

Heron, J. (1973) *Experiential Training Techniques*, Human Potential Research Project, University of Surrey, Guildford, Surrey.

Heron, J. (1989) *Facilitators' Manual*, Kogan Page, London.

Tuckman, B. (1965) Developmental sequences in small groups, *Psychological Bulletin*, **63**, no. 6, 384–99.

Whittington, D.S. (1987) *Using Groups To Help People*, Tavistock/Routledge, London.

Skills Check: Part Two

Sit quietly and reflect on the skills that have been discussed in this section. How many of them are applicable in your health care setting? To what degree do you feel that you have had training in those that are applicable?

Now ask yourself the following questions:

- What do I need to do to enhance my therapeutic skills?
- Am I an effective listener?
- If not, what gets in the way of my listening effectively?
- Am I an effective counsellor?
- What degree of structure do I use in counselling?
- If I were asked to facilitate a group tomorrow, what would I have to do now?

PART THREE
Organizational Skills

INTRODUCTION

All health care professionals work in organizations. Many find themselves faced with a managerial function at some point. In Part Three, various organizational skills are explored.

Chapter 7 identifies some of the specific skills that arise in management: managing time and people, delegation and appraisal. In Chapter 8, a range of skills to do with running and organizing meetings is considered. Many people loathe meetings and see them as a waste of time. How best can they be used to ensure that *everyone* benefits? How best can they be organized to ensure that nobody's time is wasted? All health professionals need a range of strategies for coping with meetings.

In the final chapter in this section, the question of interviewing is addressed. Again, most health professionals find that they have to organize and set up interviews — often as part of the appointment process. The other side to the issue of interviewing is *being interviewed.* In Chapter 9 the process of being a candidate at an interview is also addressed and the chapter closes with details of how to write and maintain a Curriculum Vitae (CV).

PART THREE

Organizational Skills

7

Management skills

Aims of the chapter

The following issues and skills are discussed in this chapter:

- managing time
- managing people
- delegation

Part of being a health professional is managing people and time. This chapter explores some aspects of management with particular emphasis on structuring time and managing work.

MANAGING TIME

The first aspect of managing your time is observing how you use it. The best way to do this is to keep a log or journal which identifies what you do and how long it takes you. A simple format for this is as follows. Fill in your log for one week.

	Task	Time Started	Time Finished
1.			
2.			
3.			
4.			

The table is self-explanatory. In it, you note every aspect of your working day: what you do and how long it takes to do it. This exercise alone can help you to identify those tasks that are lengthy in execution. This may help you to reorganize what you do and plan your time more effectively. What the log also helps you to do is to identify *inefficiencies* in your use of time. As you map out your day, you become aware of how time is wasted though bad planning.

The next stage is to identify your main objectives. The log should help you to see what tasks you carry out most frequently. The point now is to identify what you *need* to do most urgently. Look through your log and try to identify the sorts of task you do in a week, then set down the three most important tasks for next week. Now, fill in a timetable for the week, mapping in, first, those three important tasks. An example of an outline timetable might be as follows:

Time	Monday	Tuesday	Wednesday	Thursday	Friday
9.00– 10.00					
10.00– 11.00					
11.00– 12.00					
12.00– 13.00	lunch	lunch	lunch	lunch	lunch
13.00– 14.00					
14.00– 15.00					
15.00– 16.00					

There are certain features to bear in mind when drawing up a timetable of this sort. First, account for each *hour* of your time at work. If you do not, you will not get an accurate picture of your use of time. Second, be realistic about your time allocation to the tasks you have planned but do not be overgenerous to yourself.

Having filled in the important tasks for the week, begin to sketch in the others. An important point, is only to programme yourself up to 60% of your time. Allow yourself 'travelling time' between tasks. Also allow yourself some free time. If you 'book' free time in this way, you are more likely to take it. If you do not, you will find things to fit the time that you have at your disposal. Also, when you work with the timetable, stick to the timings as far as possible. If you find that an appointment runs short of the time you have allowed, make a note of the fact and give yourself some extra free time. Do not bring forward an appointment unless absolutely necessary. If you do, you will not be able to monitor your use of time so accurately. Work with your new timetable for another week.

During the time that you use the timetable, you will begin to see patterns forming. Where did you underestimate? Where did you allow too much time? How long did you spend doing paper-work that was unexpected? Had you allowed for things like opening mail and writing reports? Also, was your day punctuated with your making 'phone calls? If so, consider programming some time into each day which you allocate as 'telephone time', then try to do all your phoning in that time. This sounds a simple solution to a difficult problem but it is surprising how much time can be saved by dealing with most of your calls in one period.

If you take a lot of incoming calls, consider using an answer-phone machine. During busy periods, have the answerphone on at all times and answer the calls that are left in a batch (during your telephone time). Clearly, whether or not you can do this will depend on the sort of work you can do. If you deal with numerous non-urgent calls, this may save you valuable time.

If you find that you are grossly under- or overestimating time allocation to a particular task, log the time taken for that task alone. The following grid can help here.

With this grid, you note down the time when the task starts and the time that you estimate it will take. On completion of the task, you jot down the actual time that was taken. In the final column, you write the reason for the under- or overestimation. In this way, you carefully monitor your work and your use of time. Once you have mastered your estimation of time more accurately, you can return to your timetable.

105

Date				
Time	Estimated Time	Actual Time	Activity	Why?

The other way of monitoring your time is to keep a TO DO list. These are widely available as pre-printed pads but the following example shows you how to draw one up on scrap paper:

	TO DO LIST
Order	Task
2.	See Mrs H.
4.	Drop suit in cleaners
3.	Attend support group if possible.
1.	Write report for P.K.

The important thing with the TO DO list is to get used to using it quickly and to keep using it. Do not allow it to become a time-wasting exercise itself. I once worked with a colleague who seemed to spend the day drawing up new and revised TO DO lists, seemingly to the exclusion of other work.

Godefroy and Clark (1989) suggest the following points for ensuring that you manage your time effectively:

- Programme no more than ten items per day,
- Divide complex and demanding tasks into more easily programmable sub-activities,
- Learn to make an accurate estimate of the time needed for each task,
- Be ambitious, but don't overload yourself,
- Programme only 60% of your time,
- Revise your plan regularly,
- Finish each task before going on to the next.

Their last item is an important one. It is easy to get caught up in what has been called the 'busy syndrome' (Bond, 1986) in which you are so swamped by things to do that you only half do a number of tasks. This causes you further anxiety and further work and leads, in turn, to greater inefficiency. Somtimes it is just a question of taking a deep breath and making a start on the pile!

Before you go any further, look through the following list of factors that may stop you organizing your time effectively and identify the ones that particularly apply to *you*.

- I don't identify priorities.
- I don't have long- and short-term goals.
- I tend to say 'Yes' to everyone.
- I don't organize my day.
- I keep two diaries.
- I don't keep a diary at all.
- I lack motivation.
- I feel stressed.
- I am burntout.
- I spend too much time on the phone.
- I spend too much time with particular clients/patients.
- I avoid the things I don't like doing.
- I take very long breaks.
- I usually arrive late.
- I take a long time to 'come round' in the morning.
- I often do useless tasks.
- I take on other people's work.
- I rewrite reports very frequently.
- I write long letters.
- I always have someone else check my work.
- I like to discuss what I do before I do it.

- I don't have the equipment I need to do the job.
- I like meeting other people, socially, during work time.
- I can't concentrate for long periods.

Once you have read through this list, add some of your own factors to it. Then act on the extended list.

MANAGING PEOPLE

The key to successful management in the health services is the management of people. There are now large numbers of easy-to-read books about people management available in the shops. In this section, the main aim is to get you to think about the way that you interrelate to the people you work with in your particular health care setting. Good social skills and the ability to listen to other people seem crucial here, as does the need to be appropriately assertive. As a means of thinking about your own skills in managing people, consider the following questions:

- How do you greet your colleagues when you meet them?
- How do you address them when you talk to them?
- How approachable are you?
- Do colleagues come to you with their personal as well as work-related problems?
- What do you imagine other people think of your work?
- Are you able to ask them?
- Do they see you as 'the boss' or as a 'colleague'?
- Do you consciously cultivate a management style?
- What do you do when you are angry with other people?
- How do you handle other people's distress?
- How do you manage the breaking of bad news?
- Do you think carefully before you discuss things with your colleagues?
- How much of what other people do is negotiable with them?
- Do you believe in letting other people do what they want?
- Do you think that you should 'manage' other people?
- Would you say that your style was 'directive' or 'person-centred'?
- How did you *learn* the style that you use?
- How could you be more effective with other people?
- Do you know your weak spots?

- Would you say that you are defensive?
- Do you encourage other people?
- Do others take part in most decisions that are made?

Considering these questions can help you to decide on what changes (if any) you need to make to your style of helping and managing others. You may want to think, too, about your own training and development. It is easy in a management position to be so caught up with the management process and with encouraging other people that your own needs and wants are overlooked. Think about two aspects to such training: formal educational courses (such as diploma courses and courses such as the Master of Business Administration) and one-off short courses or study days. The former can help in the long term to make you more effective in your work. The latter can be great morale boosters and motivators.

DELEGATION

Unless they work in a very small team and are part of a well-defined organization and structure, most managers need to delegate. Many managers, however, are not particularly good at delegation. As a simple rule of thumb, the following questions can help to identify the areas of work that can be delegated. Try to answer them now:

- What do you *have* to do?
- What do others *have* to do?
- What are you doing at present that others *could* do?
- What are you doing at present that others might *do better*?

Through writing notes about the nature of your work and the work of others that you supervise, it becomes clearer how best to allocate work fairly to other people. Clearly, it is important that you do not delegate all of your work to others. Nor should you dodge those tasks that are unpleasant and yet which *should* be carried out by you. Also, it is essential that your staff are not overloaded with work and that work is fairly and reasonably allocated. At this point you might want to reflect on the degree to which you appreciate the workload of those with whom you work — at this moment. Do you have difficulty in recalling who does what? Are you unclear about how many tasks other colleagues are engaged in? Part of the process of successful delegation is making sure that you are asking the right person to carry out the task. The subset of that issue is the degree to which you understand and appreciate the nature of the job that that person is doing at present. Here are some reasons for *not* delegating:

- I want the thanks for a particular task. This is a fairly egotistical reason for not delegating and one associated, perhaps, more frequently with a younger or newer manager. Part of the process of managing is to encourage others to develop both personally and within the organization.
- I know what needs to be done. Others will, too, if you allow them the chance.
- I don't want mistakes made. Again, people who are trusted to work and find out solutions to problems are more likely to be better decision makers in the future. An organization which encourages some 'mistake making' is likely to be a healthy one. Most people learn, to some degree, from their mistakes.
- People may not want to do the things that I delegate to them. But this is why you are a manager. Your task is to 'sell' ideas to others and also to be assertive enough to ask them to do those things that they may not want to.
- I want to be popular. You will be more popular if you are seen to be assertive, fair and consistent. You will not be particularly popular if you are seen as the person who takes on everything yourself and delegates nothing.

The following issues are important once you have decided to delegate:

- Be clear about *what* you are delegating. Is it a task or is it also the responsibility that goes with that task?
- Set a time limit. Expect that people work better when they are clear about how much time they have to complete a task. Be realistic about the amount of time you allocate.
- Be sure the other person knows what has been delegated. Be sure, too, that they know whether or not responsibility for the task has also been delegated.
- Be available if help is required but do not constantly check on progress.

SUMMARY OF THE CHAPTER

Managing time and managing people are two key elements in the communication system of any organization. This is as true in the health professions as it is in business. This chapter has explored practical ways to enhance your time and people skills.

REFERENCES

Bond, M. (1986) *Stress and Self-Awareness*, Heinemann, London.
Godefroy, C.H. and Clark, J. (1989) *The Complete Time Management System*, Piatkus, London.

8

Meeting skills

Aims of the chapter

The following skills and issues are discussed in this chapter:

- identifying types of meetings
- planning the meeting
- the agenda
- running the meeting
- coping with contingencies
- notes and minutes

Health professionals are required to attend and run numerous meetings. Why do *you* go to meetings? What sorts of meetings do you go to? What are their functions? Before anything else happens, it is essential to know what *sort* of meeting you are being asked to organize, plan and run.

Williams (1984) identifies six main sorts of meetings:

1. Command meeting. This is the meeting called by a manager to pass on information or to exercise control over staff. This sort of meeting may be a common one in the health professions.
2. Selling meeting. In this sort of meeting, an individual or group of people are engaged in trying to convince others of a need or of the validity of a planned project.
3. Advisory meeting. This meeting is called to exchange ideas or information or to seek opinions.
4. Negotiating meeting. Here the object is to reach a compromise or agreement over a matter or matters in some dispute. This type of meeting may be called when there are changes being brought about in an organization or where job roles are changing.

5. Problem-solving meeting. This is a meeting called to tackle a specific problem or series of problems that face a group of health professionals or an organization.
6. Support meeting. Here people meet to help each other, to offer support and, often, to express feelings and emotions. Such meetings are often organized by or for relatives or those suffering in particular life situations.

Whilst this may not be an exhaustive classification of all possible types of meetings, it is clear that the *aims* of a particular meeting will depend upon that meeting's purpose. As a variety of issues regarding group facilitation and therapy have been addressed already in this book (and also in later chapters), the types of meeting methods discussed in this chapter are to do with more *formal* meetings. Thus, the sorts of meetings that will require the skills described in this chapter are more likely to be the command, negotiating and problem-solving ones.

PLANNING THE MEETING

Having decided what sort of meeting you want to call, there are other considerations to make. A short list of these would be:

- Who needs to be at the meeting? This is not always as easy to answer as it might seem. It is tempting to invite the whole department to every meeting. Think about this carefully and only invite the essential people.
- Where will the meeting be held? Is the room that you have in mind large enough or even too large? Do you have to book ahead to make sure that the room is available?
- What is the *purpose* of the meeting? Your meeting, might, for example, be called for any of the following purposes:
  - information giving,
  - obtaining information,
  - creating and sharing ideas,
  - departmental decision making,
  - patient/client policy making,
  - presenting proposals,
  - questioning other people's proposals,
  - discussing patient/client progress.

113

- How will you inform people of the meeting? One frequent cry amongst health professionals is that they did not know that a meeting was to be held.
- Who will chair the meeting? Godefroy and Clark (1989) suggest the following method of selecting a chairman if the issue has not been resolved prior to the meeting. Once the meeting is in session, you count up to three. At three, each participant points to another. The person with the most votes is elected to the chair. The rest of this chapter, however, anticipates that *you* will be the chairman.

AGENDA

It is very frustrating to arrive at a meeting to find that no agenda has been set. Set it well in advance of the meeting. If necessary, phone or circulate a list to colleagues for agenda items. Then draw up a list of priorities. It may help if you think in terms of:

- What *must* be on the agenda;
- What *should* be on the agenda;
- What *could* be on the agenda.

The *must* items will naturally go straight on the final agenda. After that, it is a question of allocating time to each item and deciding what can go on it from what is left on your list. The point of this sort of planning is that it can help you focus very clearly on how much time you spend on items in the meeting itself. A little forethought can pay great dividends.

RUNNING THE MEETING

Think carefully about how you will run your meeting. First, start exactly on time and do not be too friendly and accepting towards latecomers. This tends to reinforce two things: first, it makes it appear that timing is not particularly important to you. Second, it gives the appearance of sloppiness. If you cannot be seen to be working to time at the beginning of the meeting, can you be trusted to work through the agenda and finish on time?

Work through your prepared agenda, keeping fairly rigidly to the time scale that you worked out when you wrote it. If you feel that you are unlikely to get through the whole agenda, negotiate changes as the need arises. This is not, however, a particularly good policy. If you can, stick to the agenda.

Pay close attention to what each person has to say, whilst keeping up a 'wide sweep' of attention to the other members of the meeting. Make sure that everyone gets a hearing and that they are satisfied with the responses that they invoke. Be prepared to sum up some of the longer comments and check with the person who has spoken to make sure that your summary is accurate. Be wary, however, of allowing the person a 'second breath', during which they repeat what they have said before.

Bring things to a clear conclusion and make sure that at the end of each item, the *action* element of a decision is noted. Make sure that no-one is unclear about their responsibilities after the meeting. Whilst all decisions will be minuted, those minutes will not be read until later. People need to leave a meeting knowing what is expected of them.

COPING WITH CONTINGENCIES

Not all meetings run to plan. A variety of ploys can be used by people at meetings, either consciously or otherwise, to disrupt the proceedings. The following issues have been identified as common 'disrupters':

- Late arrival. Here, one member of the meeting arrives late and takes some time to settle. There is usually considerable shuffling of papers and moving of seats as the person sits down. One way to counteract this behaviour is to insist on people arriving on time. Another is to ask the late arriver to take his or her place quickly so as minimally to disrupt the meeting. If the behaviour persists from meeting to meeting, the chairman may have to talk to the late arriver, away from the meeting.
- Pairing. Here, two members of the meeting quietly collude with each other. Sometimes they speak almost sub-vocally to each other and make 'asides' about other members of the meeting. Another behaviour associated with pairing is note passing between two people sitting together. It is, perhaps, a sign of regression and can be a direct threat to the chair. Sometimes, though, it is a sign of boredom and the chairman

who encounters a lot of pairing should reconsider the length or number of meetings that are held.

- Walking out. One fairly legitimate reason for a member to walk out is that they have a prior engagement elsewhere. Consider, though, why this is happening. Has the meeting run on too long? Did it start late and is it now running late? If so, remedial action needs to be taken in the future. Alternatively, the person may *plan* to leave early, thus bringing the meeting's attention to him or herself. As with other such manoeuvres, the chairman may have to talk to this person away from the meeting. More difficult to handle is the person who walks out of the meeting in an emotionally charged state. This contingency must be dealt with in context. Sometimes it is appropriate to ask someone to follow them and talk to them. At other times, it is better merely to allow the person to leave. It is rarely a good idea to abandon the meeting, although a short 'cooling off' break may be appropriate.

- Delaying. Here, one or more members take time over small issues that everyone else feels could be dealt with more rapidly. It is important to discriminate between delaying and appropriate attention to detail. It should not be assumed that all detailed questioning and discussion is symptomatic of delaying.

- The Straw Person Syndrome. This is a special case of delaying. Here, a detail 'case' is built up by one or more of the meeting members — a case that has little evidence or relevance. An example of how such straw man arguments starts is as follows:

  'Supposing if some of our case workers are taken out of the department and then we are all rehoused. Supposing, then, that the government changes its policy on hospital admissions and then we find ourselves short of staff . . .'

  The point about the straw man argument is that it uses so many 'ifs' that the picture that is painted is usually almost completely unrelated to likelihood or reality. Sometimes in the debate that follows, the straw man debater uses the 'Yes but . . .' ploy (Berne, 1974). To every objection to his or her argument, he or she says something like 'Yes, but what happens if . . .'. One way of coping with such a scenario is gently to unpack the person's argument with logic and invitations to address the *likelihood* of the scenario. The straw person syndrome is not always easy to deal with and is yet another variety of delaying tactic.

- Overtalking. Some people like to make themselves heard at meetings. Others like to take over the meeting. The 'over-talker' must be differentiated from the person who has a particular interest in the topic on the agenda. The overtalker usually has to say more than anyone else on *every* topic. Such a person needs firm direction from the chair and it is here that the chair may want to direct the order of speaking, thus: 'Sarah, first, then Peter . . .'.

NOTES AND MINUTES

It is important to establish early on in the proceedings who will take the minutes of the meeting. Whilst some chairpersons may prefer this to be a voluntary task, it is important that the chairperson does not find him- or herself doing the job, whilst trying to chair the meeting. It may be preferable, if possible, to take on secretarial help here. It is vital that whoever takes the minutes, has either had experience of such minute taking or has a clear idea of how to lay them out once they are taken.

Finally, the issue of how or whether to take personal notes during a meeting. If the meeting is properly minuted, detailed notes should not be necessary. However, it is important that everyone brings their diaries to meetings in order to set the times and dates of future meetings. It is usually better to set such times and dates for at least the next three meetings. Also, members who are voted or delegated certain tasks away from the meeting and before the publication of the minutes may want to jot down the elements that are involved in those tasks.

Two methods of notetaking can be recommended. First is the style which makes use of separate 'blocks' of works. This method is illustrated below. The advantage of this method is that it makes it immediately clear where one note finishes and the next one starts. It is also a very easy method to get used to and many people use it for notetaking in educational settings.

Notetaking Style One

1. Starting tomorrow, all staff will have to draw up personal plans for coping with emergencies. These should include the following:

- Date and time
- Name(s)
- Nature of the emergency
- Who reported to
- Other action taken

Remember to work on this tonight and draft out plan.

2. Peter is to take on the role of team leader in the psychiatric division. All psychiatric referrals should be made through him in the future. How will this affect Sarah and David? Discuss this with them pronto!

3. New Green Paper to be distributed through the department. Advised to read the sections on changes in child care. It may be worth getting a copy of this. Ring bookshop tomorrow or consider library copy. Will the students need a session on this?

The second style of notetaking is the well-known 'spider's web' method. Here, a central theme is jotted down in the middle of the notepad. Then, 'spokes' are developed out of the central theme and 'branches' added to the spokes. The advantage of this method is that it allows you to write as you think. It also allows you to take in a wide range of details in one go. The disadvantage is that such notetaking often looks untidy and this may upset tidy people. An example of this style is illustrated below. The style is also widely used in education and learning settings.

Notetaking Style Two

Finally, it is important to file such notes. It is worth considering keeping a 'meetings file' in the form of a ring binder divided into sections for each of the meetings that you go to or chair. Even more organized is to have one file for meetings that you chair and another for those where you are a member. If you keep such

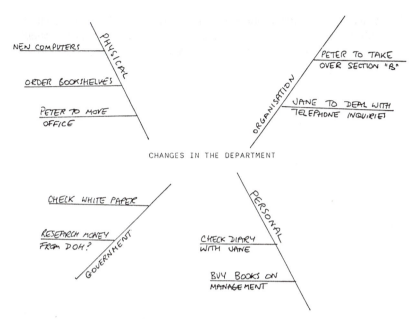

CHANGES IN THE DEPARTMENT

files, you can take them with you to each meeting and make reference to previous agenda and prior notetaking. This tends to be a much better approach than merely dropping all of your notes and agenda into a file in a filing cabinet. As we have noted throughout this chapter, the key element in effective meeting management is *structure*. Structure in notetaking and filing will also pay off in making better use of your time and resources.

SUMMARY OF THE CHAPTER

This chapter has discussed skills related to running a variety of meetings but *particularly* the more formal chaired meeting. By its nature, the chaired meeting is highly structured. You are advised to use that structure to make your meetings productive. The structure can also give you confidence when the going gets rough.

REFERENCES

Berne, E. (1974) *Games People Play*, Penguin, Harmondsworth.
Godefroy, C.H. and Clark, J. (1989) *The Complete Time Management System*, Piatkus, London.

9

Interview skills

Aims of the chapter

The following skills and issues are discussed in this chapter:

- selection
- conducting the interview
- decision making
- being interviewed
- preparing a curriculum vitae (CV)

SELECTION

The first stage in setting up the process of selection interviews is the placing of advertisements. First, define your post, then write the advert. What you must be clear about is what the job entails and what sort of people you want applying for it. Once you have done that, it is important to make sure that all of the information that a prospective employee will want is in the advertisement when it appears. Issues include:

- the job title,
- a short summary of what the job involves,
- the salary scale,
- who may apply,
- to whom they might apply (along with an address and 'phone number).

Whilst it is easy to be overinclusive in advertisements, it is also possible to be too frugal. Consider, too, the 'tone' of the advertisement. Try to avoid overly formal language. An example of a stilted and formal tone might be:

Suitably Qualified Applicants are Invited to Apply for The Post of:

Senior Nurse

Applicants with a recent history of successful management in acute settings will be considered for the above post. The following are essential for this post:

- Registration on the General Part of the Register,
- A minimum of three years experience in a post of charge nurse or above,
- Willingness to study for a degree or higher degree.

Suitable applicants may apply, in the first instance, to Mr P. Davies, Senior Personnel Officer, Brigemont General Hospital, Brigemont, Somerset. Phone: 0657-3434 Ext. 231

Consider ways that such an advert could be made more appealing. First of all, try to avoid ambiguous and superfluous phrases such as 'suitably qualified applicants' (are unsuitably qualified ones likely to apply?) and 'with a recent history of' (this sounds as thought the applicants might be expected to have a *medical* history) and 'in the first instance' (what exactly *does* this mean?). Also, consider offering your candidates the full name of the person that they can contact (Peter Davies) and recommend that they can contact him for an informal visit. Generally try to be welcoming in your approach to advertisement writing. Remember that your advertisement helps to form the first impression that people have of your organization. People other than job applicants read adverts too.

SHORTLISTING

It is usual for shortlisting to be carried out by a panel of people. It is often best for this process to be chaired and to be run along fairly structured lines. First, the shortlisting group draws up a list of criteria for the job. Once agreed upon, it is a relatively simple clerical task to work through the applications and screen out those applications that do not qualify against those criteria. In the second round, detailed discussion and reading of application forms can take place to determine the final shortlist. It is useful if each person draws up a list of three people that they would like to see interviewed and then, in turn, each person justifies the three that they have chosen. From this process, the final list is devised.

The other consideration, before interviewing, is then the question of whether or not references are taken up prior to interviewing. Once that decision has been made, the next is to determine whether or not those references will be *read* by the interviewing panel before the interviews. Some panels prefer to interview first and read the references after they have settled on one or two possible candidates for the job.

THE INTERVIEW

Some people loathe the prospect of interviewing almost as much as they do the process of being interviewed. A little careful planning can help here. Considerations that need to be made prior to the interview are these:

- Where will the interviewees gather and who will meet them to settle them there?
- Who will call the interviewee and will that person then introduce them to each member of the panel?
- How will the interview proceed? A traditional approach is for each of the interviewers to ask two or three questions of each person (usually the same questions). This method of interview does not allow for any real interaction between interviewer and interviewee. A more imaginative approach is to allocate a certain amount of time to each interviewer and to allow them to develop a rapport and discussion with the interviewee.
- Who will invite the interviewee to ask questions at the end of the interview and who will round off the process and thank the candidate for coming?
- What will be the standard response to when the outcome of the interview will be made known to interviewees?

If these issues can be decided upon through discussion, prior to the interview, the whole process can be more successful. Also, if the interview panel is to be a large one, it is important that it is chaired. The chairperson might be a contributing interviewer or may be a person who limits their interaction to the chairing process.

It is helpful if the interview also follows a reasonably formal structure, even if the discussion during the interview is fairly unstructured. Typically, the following points are covered during a job interview:

- The applicants' account of their education and work prior to the application;
- Reasons for wanting the job;
- Strengths and weaknesses;
- Special factors that the applicant can bring to the post;
- Financial and logistic issues (when the applicant would be able to start work, entry on the salary scale, etc.).

Ideally, the interview should be a two-way process. Not only does the interview panel interview the applicant but the applicant also has the chance to discuss the job and his or her suitability for it. The more formal the interview, the less the likelihood of a productive discussion occurring. If only highly structured questions are asked, only 'best performance' answers will be offered. Remember that the candidate is likely to have rehearsed most of the standard interview questions prior to this moment. The more informal, open-ended interviews (within a more formal outer structure) are more likely to yield in-depth answers and insights.

Most people who have conducted interviews are familiar with the idea of starting the interview with a few simple questions to get the candidate talking. These usually relate to travelling to the interview or to the candidates' familiarity with the area. It is useful to notice the candidates' 'body language' or non-verbal aspects of communication and to time the 'deeper' and more penetrating questions with visible signs of relaxation. Indicators, here, may be:

- Uncrossing of previously crossed arms and legs;
- Increased levels of eye contact;
- Smiling;
- Increased use of hand gestures;
- Change in depth of breathing;
- Change of tone in voice.

During the 'body' of the interview, it is helpful if all questions are clear, unambiguous and contain only *one* question. It is easy, for example, to find yourself asking the following sort of multiple question:

'How do you cope with stress? Do you find that you can relax fairly easily after work? Or are you a person who tends to take their work home with them? What are your views on this?'

Four questions in one. Instead, make sure that you are relaxed and clear about what it is you want to ask. Then ask *one* clear question. Follow up that question with a series of 'open' questions, if necessary, to encourage further discussion. Examples of open questions include:

'What did you do then . . . ?'
'How do you feel about that . . . ?'
'Can you think of other examples . . . ?'
'What do you think of that . . . ?'
'How do you do that . . . ?'

All of these open questions should be asked in a supportive and caring manner and not in an inquisitorial way. The aim is for both you and the interviewee to get to know each other better. Remember that the person you are interviewing also has to make a decision about whether or not she or he wants to work with you and your colleagues. As an interviewer, you are saying a lot about the organization in which you work.

When the interviewee is answering your questions, make sure that you listen. It is easy when you are anxious to be caught up with your own questions to the point that you no longer listen to the answers. An aid to the listening process is suggested by Egan (1990) who offers the following pointers to effective listening behaviour (these are discussed in greater detail in Chapter 4 of this book):

- Sit squarely: face the interviewee rather than sit next to them,
- Sit in an 'open' position and try not to fold your arms and legs as this suggests defensiveness,
- Lean slightly towards the other person,
- Maintain reasonable eye contact,
- Relax and resist the temptation to rehearse future questions while you are listening to the interviewee's answers.

DECISION MAKING

Once you have interviewed all of the candidates, the decision has to be made as to whom you appoint. The option usually exists, too, to decide whether or not you *do* appoint. The factors that will help you in this process are:

- Notes that you have taken after each interview. It is not a good plan to make notes *during* the interview, at least not if you are asking the questions. It is sometimes reasonable for those not asking the questions to take notes.
- Discussion evolving out of a 'round' conducted at the end of the interviews. In this activity, each interviewer, in turn, says who they felt to be the best two candidates and why. No further discussion occurs until each person has spoken.
- Re-reading (or reading for the first time, as appropriate) of the references.

It is usually a good idea to submit all decisions to a 'devil's advocate' process in which likely candidates are explored through the question of 'why they should not be appointed' as well as through the more usual one of 'why they should be appointed'. This allows for clarity of decision making and the covering of most of the issues governing appointment.

BEING INTERVIEWED

The other side of the interview process is that of being interviewed. As noted above, it is by no means clear which aspect of the process is the more anxiety making. Some people find the business of conducting interviews very traumatic. It is this factor that can help you to overcome your own preinterview nerves — the interviewers are quite likely to be nervous.

PRESENTING YOURSELF

There are certain fairly simple things that you can do to ensure that you are seen in your best light. These include the following:

- Make sure that the interviewers have what they asked for. Ensure that your application form or introductory letter is complete. If you are asked to present a CV, make sure that it is properly filled out. How to prepare a CV and what to put in it is described later in this chapter.

- Do your homework. Know something about the organization in which you are being interviewed. If possible, always make an informal (although scheduled) visit, prior to the interview but do not make this visit on the same day as the interview.

- Practise the interview process with a colleague or friend. Ask that person to field you a number of difficult questions and anticipate your answers. Practise answering questions with concise but accurate answers. On the one hand, no interviewer wants you to be monosyllabic, on the other, interviewers tend not to like having to interrupt you so that they can get on with the next question.

- Look your best. It is usually best to dress reasonably formally (but not flashily) for interviews. It is a mistake to think that people a) do not notice clothes, b) should accept you for what you are or c) no longer take clothes and appearance into consideration. Spend some time thinking about how you will look but do not spend so much time on it that you fail to relax during the interview. Do not try to stun the interview panel.

- Arrive in plenty of time. You can always stop for coffee near to the interview site. On the other hand, it is not a good plan to leave things too late. It is certainly a bad plan to arrive late. If it is inevitable that you will be late, however, 'phone through to inform the interview panel.

- Prepare some short questions that you can ask when approached by the panel. Do not ask 'impossible' questions ('Could you tell me the history of this unit?'). Keep your questions simple and make sure that they can be answered by the interviewer in a couple of sentences. If you have real anxieties about the job, make sure that these are surfaced during your questioning period. Remember from the discussion above that the interview should be a two-way process — you should be finding out about the people who are interviewing you.

Finally, make sure that you really want the job for which you are applying. Perhaps you cannot always make up your mind before you go for the interview but it is a mistake to use interviews merely as 'experience' and to go through an interview process with no intention of taking the job if you are offered it.

127

Remember that many interviewers will ask you if you *will* take the job if it is offered you.

PREPARING A CV

The CV or curriculum vitae is just that, a 'life curriculum' or description of your life to date. Think carefully about what you put in it. It is usually a good idea to keep a copy of your CV in your possession at all times and to update it regularly. That way, when you apply for a job, there is no problem in remembering what you have and have not done. If you use a computer and wordprocessor, it is useful to keep your CV as a file and to add to the file as new things happen to you. You may want to keep a 'short version' which summarizes the essential parts of your personal history, as well as the full version. The short version can be a useful aid to filling in application forms and may be asked for during applications for jobs, grants or scholarships.

CVs typically cover the following subject areas:

- Name
- Address
- Work Address
- Date of Birth
- Age
- Marital Status
- Place of Birth
- Nationality
- Current Post
- Secondary, Professional and Higher Education
- Other Professional Training (Short courses, management courses, etc.)
- Professional Employment
- Summary of Responsibilities in Present Post
- Committee Membership
- Other Professional Activities (membership of unions, clubs, associations, editorial boards, external examining, etc.)
- Other Activities (governership of schools, membership of other organizations, etc.)
- Miscellaneous Section (Driving licence, wordprocessing skills, etc.)
- Research

- Conference Papers
- Publications (Books, Chapters in Books, Articles in refereed journals, Articles in other journals)

Not all of these headings will be necessary or appropriate to everyone's CV but you should aim at making yours as comprehensive as possible. Make sure that all the dates are correct and that the spelling and layout are appropriate. At the end of the CV it is sometimes correct to include the names and addresses of two or three people who will write references for you. Make sure that you ask their permission before you do so.

SUMMARY OF THE CHAPTER

This chapter has considered the skills involved in the two sides of interviewing: the process of interviewing other people and the process of being interviewed. It has illustrated how, through simple structure, the business of applying for jobs can be made less anxiety provoking for all concerned. All of the skills described here can also be applied in other interview situations, e.g. applications for grants, scholarships and fellowships.

REFERENCES

Egan, G. (1990) *The Skilled Helper*, 4th edn, Brooks/Cole, Pacific Grove, California.

Skills Check: Part Three

Sit quietly and reflect on the skills that have been discussed in this section. How many of them are applicable in your health care setting? To what degree do you feel that you have had training in those that are applicable?

Now ask yourself the following questions:

- What am I like as a manager?
- How organized am I?
- How effectively do I use my time?
- If I were asked to chair a meeting tomorrow, what would I have to do now?

PART FOUR

Personal Skills

INTRODUCTION

There is an increasing realization amongst health professionals that we must also care for ourselves. In the final part of this book, three elements of communication skills are examined. First, in Chapter 10, the question of how to improve writing skills is addressed. Whether we are writing essays and projects of reports for a management committee, we all have to write. Many academics are also required to write for publication. This issue is also explored in this chapter.

Chapter 11 is about being assertive. Assertiveness skills are not only important for enabling us to care effectively for others, they are also the means by which our own needs are met. If our own needs are frequently ignored or bypassed we are on a course for burnout, the outcome of caring for others without our paying attention to ourselves.

The final chapter is about that which underpins all aspects of caring and communication: self-awareness. With increased self-awareness we can learn to help others by staying in touch with our own thoughts, feelings, attitudes and beliefs. The chapter identifies practical ways of enhancing such awareness.

10

Writing skills

Aims of the chapter

In this chapter, the following skills and issues are discussed:

- basic principles of writing
- keeping references
- layout
- writing for publication
- using a computer for writing larger projects

BASIC PRINCIPLES

Although health professionals face a variety of writing tasks, many of the rules of good writing apply to all. In this chapter we explore some of the principles of effective written communication. First, the accent is on identifying certain basic rules, then the focus shifts to keeping references. Any health professional who has to undertake basic or further education will be required to reference projects, essays, dissertations and reports. It pays to think a little about how such references may be recorded. In the later parts of this chapter, the discussion moves on to the layout of a written piece and then on to report writing and writing for publication. Increasingly, the route to development in the health professions, for the career-minded person, is via published work — often, although not always, in professional journals. This is, in itself, a form of communication — the communication of new ideas and of research to a wider audience.

What basic principles can be applied to all writing? A shortlist of such principles would include the following:

- Write short sentences.
- Write short paragraphs: three or four sentences is nearly always enough.
- Write to communicate, not to impress. Inflated language and extensive use of jargon rarely impresses the reader. Nor does it usually impress editors and managers.
- Avoid lengthy quotations of other people's work. Wherever possible paraphrase the writing of others, giving full acknowledgement to the original writer in the form of a reference, e.g. (Brown, 1989).
- Write like you speak. Read through what you write and ask yourself: 'would I *say* this?' If you wouldn't, think about how you could rewrite what you have written to make it more readable. People often make the mistake of thinking that 'correct' writing somehow sounds more intelligent than 'readable' writing.

KEEPING REFERENCES

As we noted in Chapter 3, most health professionals need to keep references to the books and papers that they read. The important thing is to develop a system of recording that suits you best and that you will keep going. Many people start a reference collection with good intentions only to discover that the whole thing becomes too cumbersome. As a general rule, keep the simplest records that you can but ones that will lead you straight back to the book or paper in question. The minimum that you will need to record for each item is:

- the name of the author
- the year of publication
- the title of the book or paper
- the publisher (if it is a book) or the name of the journal (if it is a paper)

Many people collect their references in a simple card file. Such files are readily available at stationers as are the cards that go with them. Also available are index cards to keep them in order. It is usually better to choose the 8″ × 5″ cards which allow for more detail to be recorded. A useful layout for a bibliographic reference card is this:

Author(s):	Year of Publication
Title:	
Publisher or name and details of journal:	
Location:	
Comments: Keywords:	

This card is then completed and filed alphabetically under author. In the comments section, it is possible to record keywords for cross-referencing the item with other items and to save important quotes. A completed card looks like this:

Smith, P.	1990
Stress in Communication	
Davis and Jones, London	
Location: Cardiff Central Library	
Comments: This has a useful review of theories of stress. Takes a 'biological' view of stress rather than a psychological one. 'Talk of stress is endemic in the health professions. It is as though the concept was quite new and necessarily dangerous' (p. 16). Keywords: Stress, psychology, life sciences	

Card files are not the only way of recording references. Some people prefer to keep them in an index book. This is rather like a home telephone directory with index pages sticking out of the side. As new references are found, they are written into the appropriate section and alphabetically, by author.

The other way of keeping references is to open a database on a computer. This approach has been discussed in Chapter 3. The advantage of this method is that as the list of references becomes larger, the computer database allows you instant access to particular items or sets of items. For example, you may want to find all of your references under the heading of 'psychology'. Whilst you could work through each of your cards and pull out all the appropriate ones, the computer database can do it for you almost instantaneously. It can also help you to prepare reference lists at the ends of essays, projects, dissertations, theses and books.

LAYOUT

Any writing that you do needs to be organized. The time to think about such organization is before you start the writing. One of the most effective means of planning any writing project is through the use of *outlining*, which can be divided into three stages.

Stage One: Brainstorming

In this stage, you write down at random any thoughts, ideas, hunches that you have about the writing project. Nothing is banned at this stage. The aim is to produce as many ideas as you can. Many you will not use in the project itself but, at this stage, the more varied and even bizarre the better. The odder ideas can lead on to more practical ones. Once you have filled a page with jottings of ideas in this way, you identify the ones that you will keep and strike out the others. Then, you look for 'patterns' in the ideas that remain and group them together. Finally, you move on to the next stage, the stage of beginning to organize your ideas more formally.

Stage Two: Identifying key headings

Having identified some groups of ideas, the next task is to find headings for those groups. Those headings then serve as the sections of your project. It is helpful to aim at between five and ten headings, whatever the nature of the project. If you are writing an essay, the ten can be ten themes that you address. If you are writing a book, the ten can be ten chapters.

Stage Three: Identifying sub-headings

Next, you carefully work through the list of headings and fill in the sub-headings and possibly, the sub-sub-headings. It is rarely useful to break up your work into more than three sets of headings. Once you have completed this stage, all that remains is to allocate a word limit to each heading and sub-heading and then to write out the body of the text.

The whole process of outlining in this way is speeded up with the use of a wordprocessing package on a computer, then the headings and sub-headings can be moved around at will and new headings and sub-headings added as necessary. There are also outlining programs specially written for this purpose. An excellent one that is released as shareware (Chapter 3) is called 'PC Outline.' It allows you to generate as many ideas as you wish and then to organize them into a range of hierarchies, at will. Alternatively, you may find the whole process more easily carried out with an A4 pad and a pen.

WRITING FOR JOURNALS

Many health professionals write for journals and magazines. Many more do not. A number of people think that they could never get anything they wrote accepted for publication. On the other hand, others feel that an essay they have written for a course might make a good published article. It might but there are better ways of doing things.

Writing for journals and magazines involves ensuring that you are very familiar with the publication you are writing for. So the first stage in getting into print is selecting the right journal. There are two approaches to the second stage. Some people feel that it is best to write a letter to the editor outlining the proposed article. Others feel it is best to send off the manuscript and to let the editor decide on its strengths and weaknesses. I think the second way works better. The letter approach takes up more time and you may be asked to write a paper that is quite different from the one you had in mind.

On the other hand, if you choose to send the manuscript off directly, you must make sure that it *exactly* fits the requirements of that journal. All professional journals publish 'instructions to authors' — most at the back of each copy. Follow these to the letter. If you slip up on any one of the requirements, many journals will simply return your manuscript. Therefore, if the instructions ask for two manuscript copies, double line spaced, on one side of A4 paper, send just that. Also send a covering letter stating that what you are sending is original and has not been offered to any other journal.

Never send duplicate copies of a manuscript to a variety of journals. What will you do if it is accepted by two? Also, some journals do not send out proofs for checking by the author. In this case, you would stand to risk the same paper being published in two journals. Attractive as it may sound, this is a sure way of encouraging editors never to take your work again.

When you send a manuscript off to a referred journal, it will be sent 'blind' to one or more professional referees. 'Blind' here refers to the fact that your name will not be on the manuscript when the referees receive it. That way, they cannot be prejudiced by knowing your name.

After the referees or the editors have made a decision, you may be asked to rewrite part of the paper. If you are asked to do this, do it exactly in the way that has been suggested. The reviewers and the editor, in this case, know best. Also, make the alterations as quickly and as accurately as you can.

Alternatively, your manuscript may be accepted outright. With acceptance may come a letter offering you a fee on publication of the article. You can haggle over this figure but it is best to accept it in the early stages of your writing career. If you have submitted your work to a referred journal, it is unlikely that you will be paid for your work but the addition of a published article in a referred journal is usually a welcomed addition to your CV.

WRITING BOOKS

Many health professionals would like to write a book or think about writing one. Whilst the whole process of book writing cannot be addressed here, the stages involved can. The secret to writing a book, particularly one that is non-fiction, is *structure*. The more organized you can be the better.

Stage One: The idea

First, you need to make sure of two things: do you have enough to say to write a book? Is there a market for what you want to write about? If you are unsure about the answer to the first, careful planning at the proposal stage can help. If the answer is then 'no', you may want to consider writing a book jointly with a colleague, partner or friend. Alternatively, you may want to edit a book written by a collection of experts, including yourself. If the answer to the second question is 'no', then it is unlikely that a publisher will give you a contract to go ahead and write the book. Notice the order here: first a contract, then the book. Do not write the book first and then try to find a publisher. You may feel that the book is very good (and, of course, it may be) but the publisher may want quite a different sort of book. The publisher, too, is much more likely to know about the market for the sort of book that you want to write.

Once you have identified exactly what it is you want to write about, contact a commissioning editor of a publisher and send them your proposal. It is reasonable practice only to submit a proposal to one publisher at a time. Also, the process of having a proposal reviewed can take some time. Most editors will send it to one or more experts in the field who then often take some time in sending back their verdict.

Stage Two: The proposal

The proposal is a vital part of the book writing process. It shows the publisher exactly what you have in mind and also helps you to organize your ideas and plan your work. Most proposals for publishers look very similar; this is a useful format:

- *Title* Whilst you may agonize over this, it need not be binding. Either you or the publisher may suggest changes at a later date.
- *Your name, qualifications, job title and address* Remember to include your phone number and offer both home and work addresses.

- *Rationale*   Here you justify the writing of the book you have in mind. Try to keep this to about two paragraphs but choose your words carefully. This section may make or break your proposal.
- *Market*   Most publishers will expect you to have identified fairly carefully the particular market that you have in mind. The process of identifying this market is also a very good way of deciding upon the 'level' that you will be writing at.
- *Comparison with other titles*   Find three or four other books in your field and write a short summary of each of them. Then write a note about how your proposed book will improve upon or supplement these books.
- *The author*   Here, you sell yourself. Write a short resumé of your professional life to date. Your main aim is to convince the editor that you are both an expert in your topic and also able to write the book.
- *Contents*   Write out the title of each of the chapters and under each offer some sub-headings to indicate the content of each. Don't forget to start with an introduction and finish with a bibliography and index.
- *Number of words and illustrations*   A fairly standard short textbook is between 50 000 and 70 000 words long. This one is about 65 000. You need to indicate your upper word limit and stick to it if you are offered a contract. Illustrations of any sort are expensive. Very few publishers will want you to include colour or monochrome photos. Some will ask you to prepare the art work for any diagrams that you include. It is best to keep diagrams and illustrations to a minimum. The cheapest sort are 'word illustrations' which show blocks of words surrounded by straight lines.
- *Date of submission of manuscript*   People write at different speeds. Even so, the publisher will want to know that you will not be writing your book forever. Given that the process of getting a contract can take some time, it is useful to suggest 'submission of manuscript one year from signing of contract' or a figure that seems reasonable and appropriate to you. A book of about 50 000 words should take between 6 months and a year to write.

Take some time over the preparation of your proposal. It is often the only thing between you and the publisher and it is the document that usually decides whether or not the company will go ahead and commission your book.

Stage Three: The contract

Once the commissioning editor has agreed to see your proposal and has received it, she will send it off for review by one or more experts on the topic. Four things can happen after this (and sometimes some considerable time after this — things do not happen quickly in the book trade).

First, the editor may write back and say that your proposal has been accepted by the company and that you will shortly be receiving a contract. This is unlikely if this is your first book.

Second, the editor may write and ask you to amend your proposal along the lines suggested by one or more of the reviewers. If this suggestion is made, make the amendments and send back the proposal.

Third, the editor may ask for a sample chapter. If this happens, take your time over it. You don't have to write the first chapter. Write the one that you are likely to be most comfortable with and write it well.

Finally (and this is the worst option) the editor may thank you for your proposal but suggest that the company cannot take it on at present. This is a polite way of saying that your proposal has been rejected. Some publishers will give you details about why it has been turned down, others will just turn it down. Either way, pick yourself up, print out a new copy of the proposal (or make modifications to it) and send it off to another publisher. If it is also rejected by them, consider writing another book. Don't give up!

If you are successful, you will be sent a formal contract to read and sign. Read it carefully and make sure that you agree with all of the clauses. If you are in doubt about anything in it, contact the editor and ask for clarification.

Stage Four: The writing

The easy part is over — now for the writing. As noted above, structure is the thing that will help in the writing of a book. You will already have planned out your chapters when you prepared the proposal. Now elaborate on those basic outlines. If you are working with a computer, open up separate files for each chapter and lay out an outline of headings and sub-headings. This will make the whole thing seem much more manageable and help to ensure that you don't repeat yourself.

Next, set yourself a plan of working. Try to write regularly and attempt to complete a certain number of words every week. If you want to be professional, write something everyday even if you don't feel like it. The discipline is good, your writing is likely to improve and you will get the book written. Remember, too, that you don't have to write the whole book in chapter order. You may decide to write the most difficult chapters first, or start with an easy one and then take on an awkward one.

However you decide to write, the three rules that apply throughout the writing process are as follows:

- be accurate
- be concise
- be consistent

Stage Five: The checking

Once you have written the first draft (and you may find it easiest to do this at speed — particularly if you are working on a computer), read through the whole manuscript, critically. Rewrite and polish as necessary. Pay particular attention to making sure that you have used short sentences and paragraphs. If possible, ask someone else to read it and to comment on it for style and readability. Finally, check all the spellings, diagrams and page numbers and references. Some of the things to *avoid* in the final read-through are these:

- spelling errors
- errors of punctuation
- repetitions of the same word in a sentence (e.g. At the centre of the town.)
- split infinitives
- long words
- sexist expressions and phrases
- clumsy and awkward phrases

Print out a final draft, double line spaced and on good quality paper. Make sure that all the pages are numbered (at this stage of the business, the publisher will refer to them as 'folios': pages refer to *printed* pages.) Have two copies made of the manuscript and send the top copy and one other to the editor.

Stage Six: The waiting

Next, the wait. If the manuscript looks as though it satisfies the contract, the editor sends it out for reading. Sometimes it will go back to one of the reviewers who read the proposal. Such reading and commenting takes time and always longer than you think. If you are asked to rewrite sections or even chapters, do so. Again, the editor is likely to know more than you about the processes of writing and publishing.

Stage Seven: the proofs

Once the manuscript has been completed, you are usually due an advance on royalties which helps to counteract some of the pain of writing. Some publishers pay an advance on the signing of contracts as well as on acceptance of the manuscript but you will have checked this before you signed the contract. Now all you have to do is wait again. This will probably be the longest wait of all. The processing of a book manuscript into a printed book is always a lengthy one. Some publishers have the pages printed in the Far East which adds even more time to the process. Eventually, though, you will see the pages of the book in proof form. Normally, you can expect to see 'page proofs'. With these, every two pages of the book are printed out onto larger sheets. You can get a good idea from these what the final book will look like.

Your task at this point is to proof read. It must be emphasized that the aim of proof reading is to find printer's errors and editing errors. It is *not* the time to make textual changes. You cannot rewrite passages of text at this stage. All that must have been completed at the manuscript stage. Major (and even minor) changes at this stage are very expensive and if you insist on changes being made you may be expected to pay for them. Check the proofs carefully.

After the proofs have been returned, or sometimes at the same time, you may be asked to compile an index. Again, this will depend on your contract. It may also depend on your preference. Some authors prefer to compile their own indexes, others are happy to have a trained indexer to do them. If you do compile your own, work quickly but accurately. Time is important at this stage and the publishers are working to tight time schedules.

Stage Eight: The publication

Then, another wait. This always *feels* the longest because you have already seen the proofs. Little compares, though, with seeing the final, completed book. Normally, your contract will allow you to claim about six complimentary copies, which may follow after the initial one. Your first copy may also arrive before publication date so don't rush out to the shops to see if it's in. Don't expect, either, that all of the bigger newspaper and bookshops will automatically stock it. Yours is likely to be a fairly specialized text so it may be stocked by the big, main bookshops and the college and university bookshops but is unlikely to be on sale at airports and railway stations. Just before publication, you will have been asked to fill in an 'author's questionnaire' which asks for details about your book, about the market and suggestions about who to notify of the book's publication. Fill this in carefully. Very often, the information in it is given to the salespeople from the publisher who will be selling the book to the bookshops. Make sure that what you write is honest but complimentary.

Once you have been through these eight stages, you may feel you want a break. Or, you may feel that you want to push ahead with another book. If you do, all you have to do is to go back to stage one and start again: the process is exactly the same.

WRITING FOR PUBLICATION WITH A COMPUTER

In Chapter 3 there was a discussion about the uses of computers in various health care related projects. Here, the aim is to identify some of the ways in which using a computer can make a direct difference to the writing of journal papers and books. Whilst not everyone adjusts to writing directly with a keyboard, the fact that a paper of a book does not have to be *rewritten* (by a copy typist) is the overriding advantage of learning to use a computer to communicate your thoughts. If you *do* decide to invest in and use a computer with a wordprocessing package, consider the following methods of making the process even easier.

- Work with the line setting set to single spacing, even though your final printout will be double spaced. If you work with single line spacing, you can see more of your work and the eye does not have to move as far to scan the words. Scrolling through documents will be faster too.

- Consider working with very wide margins whilst you are typing. This has the effect of making the screen look like this:

  The advantage of this sort of setting is that it allows you to see a lot of your work very easily. You no longer have to scan long sentences but, instead, your work is broken up into small, visible chunks.

- Try to learn *all* of the functions of your wordprocessor. It is surprising how easy life can be once you let the computer do some of the more routine tasks for you.
- If your wordprocessor supports them, make liberal use of macros (the linking of a series of keystrokes to a single set of keystrokes). Well thought-out macros can save you time when cutting and pasting, spellchecking, wordcounting and backing up your work.
- Count words regularly. Regular word counts improve the style and consistency of your work by ensuring that you stick to the word limits that you set yourself at the proposal stage.
- Put references in at a later date, if recalling them whilst writing is difficult. Simply place the following code into your writing wherever a reference should appear (***). Then, when you have finished the bulk of your writing, have the wordprocessor search for all the (***)s and insert the appropriate references as you go.
- If your wordprocessor supports them, make good use of style sheets to ensure a uniform look to written work — particularly when you are writing a longer project such as a thesis or book. Style sheets can ensure that all your chapter headings and sub-headings are identical in style.
- If you have to print out a very long document (such as the thesis or book mentioned above) on a dot matrix printer, consider printing it in bold and draft quality. This is much quicker than printing in near letter quality and looks almost as good.
- Keep long documents divided into smaller sections by having a separate file for each section. Some wordprocessors allow you to pull a number of files together so that you can view the entire project as a whole.
- Consider laying out all of your headings and sub-headings for

your entire project, before you start to type the body of the text. This will ensure uniformity of layout and you will also be encouraged by the regular appearance of sub-headings. This method also aids consistency and helps you avoid repetition.

- Despite all of these suggestions, keep your wordprocessing simple. Avoid using fancy fonts and italics. If you want to indicate italics in a manuscript for publication, stick to using the underlining function.

- For work that is to be published, avoid elaborate diagrams, particularly ones that use vertical lines. Whilst your word-processor may be able to reproduce them, such diagrams are expensive to reproduce in published work.

- Write fast and edit later. One of the main advantages of wordprocessing is the editing facility. This relieves you from having to think too hard about spelling and sentence construction in your initial drafts.

- Back up your work as a matter of course. Do not be tempted to trust your hard disc, if you have one. All hard discs fail at some time. If your wordprocessor allows it, set it to do automatic backups, while you work. Remember, though, that those backups are lost when you turn off the computer. If you are working on a large and important project, consider having at least two sets of backup discs. Keep them in two separate places: one set at home and the other at work. Remember, though, to continue to back up both sets.

- If you are writing for publication, ask your publisher if you can submit your work on disc. Some journals will accept manuscripts in this format. Most book publishers, however, will want a hard (paper) copy as well as the manuscript on disc. Submitting a work on disc can help to speed up the processing time at the publishers.

- Consider using a 'notepad' program (such as 'Sidekick'), while you work in your wordprocessor. This allows you to make quick memos to yourself as you type. Otherwise, don't be afraid to leave yourself comments as you go. Again, use the *** symbols to indicate the beginning and end of such memos and later do a search for those symbols. The two sets will tell you where the 'memo' starts and ends.

- Consider running off a copy of larger projects in 'draft' print-out mode. You can then use this to read through the entire project and you are free to scribble notes and changes all over it. A manuscript often 'reads' quite differently once it is printed out.

- Do not use headers or footers in your final manuscript. If these identify your name in a paper that is being sent out for 'blind' referring, then the editor will have to erase that name from each sheet. If you are submitting a book manuscript, the headers and footers will also have to be erased by a sub-editor. Make sure, though, that you number every page.
- If you are using a dot matrix printer for printing out a thesis or book manuscript, make sure that you have at least two spare ribbons. I tried printing out a manuscript one Sunday with one, used ribbon. By page 300, the manuscript was unreadable.

SUMMARY OF THE CHAPTER

Writing is an important aspect of communication in the health professions. This chapter has explored some of the nuts and bolts of the writing process and has examined the stages through which you must go if you are to see your written work in print. Writing for publication can be an enjoyable activity and is a vital one for anyone employed in an academic capacity within the health professions. The chapter closed with suggestions about how to speed up and improve your writing for publication with the aid of a computer.

11

Assertiveness skills

Aims of the chapter

In this chapter, the following skills and issues are discussed:

- what is assertion?
- why be assertive?
- assertiveness skills

WHAT IS ASSERTION?

We have noted that both caring and working in organizations take their toll on the individual. Sometimes the person's own needs become subsumed within the demands of the organization or profession. One positive way of coping with stress in organizations and in the caring professions is to become more assertive. Assertiveness is often confused with being aggressive — there are important differences. The assertive person is the one who can state clearly and calmly what she wants to say, does not back down in the face of disagreement and is prepared to repeat what she has to say, if necessary. Woodcock and Francis (1983) identify the following barriers to assertiveness:

1. *Lack of Practice* you do not test your limits enough and discover whether you can be more assertive,
2. *Formative Training* your early training by parents and others diminished your capacity to stand up for yourself,
3. *Being Unclear* you do not have clear standards and you are unsure of what you want,
4. *Fear of Hostility* you are afraid of anger or negative responses and you want to be considered reasonable,

Submissive Approach: (Pussyfooting)	Assertive Approach	Aggressive Approach: (Sledgehammering)
The person avoids conflict and confrontation by avoiding the topic in hand.	The person is clear, calm and prepared to repeat what she has to say.	The person is heavy-handed and makes a personal attack of the issue.

Figure 11.1 Three possible approaches to confrontation

5. *Undervaluing Yourself* you do not feel that you have the right to stand firm and demand correct and fair treatment,
6. *Poor Presentation* your self-expression tends to be vague, unimpressive, confusing or emotional.

Given that most health professionals spend much of their time considering the needs of others, it seems likely that many over-look the personal needs identified within Woodcock and Francis' list of barriers to assertiveness. Part of the process of coping with stress is also the process of learning to identify and assert personal needs and wants.

A continuum may be drawn that accounts for a range of types of behaviour ranging from the submissive to the aggressive, with assertive behaviour being the mid point on such a continuum (Figure 11.1).

Heron (1986) has argued that when we have to confront another person, we tend to feel anxiety at the prospect. As a result of that anxiety we tend either to 'pussyfoot' (and be submissive) or 'sledgehammer' (and be aggressive). So it is with being assertive. Most people when they are learning how to assert themselves experience anxiety and as a result tend to be either submissive or aggressive. Other people handle that anxiety by swinging right the way through the continuum. They start submissively, then develop a sort of confidence and rush into an aggressive attack on the other person. Alternatively, other people deal with their anxiety by starting an encounter very aggressively and quickly back off into submission. The level and calm approach of being assertive takes practice, nerve and confidence.

Consider the following examples of Heron's three types:

The pussyfooting approach

1. 'There's something I want to talk to you about . . . I don't really know how to put this . . . whatever you do, don't take offence at what I have to say . . .'
2. 'I don't expect you will like this but I think it is better that I say it than keep quiet about it . . . on the other hand, perhaps it's better to say nothing.'
3. 'I know that you have an awful lot of work and I don't want to add to it. Perhaps I ought to discuss what I have in mind with someone else.'

The sledgehammer approach

1. 'What you do annoys me. If you had any feelings at all, you wouldn't get home so late . . . but that's typical of you.'
2. 'I give up with you. I bet you don't even know what I'm upset about . . .'
3. 'Everybody round here is busy. I don't know why you think you're so special. I want you to take on another caseload.'

The assertive approach

1. 'I would prefer it if you could get home a little earlier.'
2. 'I'm feeling angry at the moment and I want to discuss our relationship.'
3. 'I would like you to consider taking on Mrs Jones and her family.'

Notice, too, in your own behaviour and that of others, that *posture* and 'body language' often have much to do with the degree to which a statement is perceived by others as submissive, aggressive or assertive. These types of postures and body statements may be described using Heron's three approaches, thus:

The pussyfooting approach

- Hunched or rounded shoulders
- Failure to face the other person directly
- Eye contact averted
- Nervous smile
- Fiddling with hands
- Nervous gestures
- Voice low pitched and apologetic

The sledgehammer approach

- Hands on hips or arms folded
- Very direct eye contact
- Angry expression
- Loud voice
- Voice threatening or angry
- Threatening or provocative hand gestures

The assertive approach

- Face to face with the other person
- 'Comfortable' eye contact
- Facial expression that is 'congruent' with what is being said
- Voice clear and calm

What is notable from these descriptions of three different approaches to confrontation is that the pussyfooting and sledgehammer approaches can have *physical* as well as psychological effects. The person who frequently adopts one of these two approaches in her dealings with others will often find that she is both physically and emotionally stressed by the experience. Becoming assertive is a potent method of learning to cope with all aspects of personal stress. It can also help to overcome *organizational* stress in that the assertive person is rather more likely to express her own needs and wants and more likely to be heard.

WHY BE ASSERTIVE?

Examples of how assertiveness can be useful include the following situations:

- when used to express the idea that a person is being asked to do too much by their employer;
- when used by a person who has never been able to express her wants and needs in a marriage;
- when used by the health professional, when facing bureaucratic processes in trying to get help for her client;
- in everyday situations in shops, offices, restaurants and other places where a stated service being offered is not actually being given;
- when used by the health professional who is attempting to modify the organizational structure of her work place.

Arguably, the assertive approach to living is the much clearer one when it comes to dealing with other human beings. The submissive person often loses friends because they come to be seen as duplicitous, sycophantic or as a 'doormat'. On the other hand, the aggressive person is rarely popular perhaps, simply because most of us don't particularly like aggression. The assertive person comes to be seen as an 'adult' person who is able to treat other people reasonably and without recourse to either childish or loutish behaviour. Hargie, Saunders and Dickson (1987) summarize the functions of assertiveness when they suggest that the appropriate use of assertive interventions can help an individual to:

1. Ensure that their personal rights are not violated.
2. Withstand unreasonable requests from others.
3. Make reasonable requests of others.
4. Deal effectively with unreasonable refusals from others.
5. Recognize the personal rights of others.
6. Change the behaviour of others towards them.

7. Avoid unnecessary aggressive conflicts.
8. Confidently and openly communicate their position on any issue. (Hargie, Saunders and Dickson, 1987)

All of these functions can enable people to reduce their stress levels in interpersonal communication. Much has been written about the topic of assertiveness and the reader is referred to the recommended reading list at the end of this volume.

Alberti and Emmons (1982) identify four major elements in assertive behaviour:

1. Intent the assertive person does not intend to be hurtful to others by stating his own needs and wants.
2. Behaviour behaviour classified as assertive would be evaluated by an 'objective observer' as honest, direct, expressive and non-destructive of others,
3. Effects behaviour classified as assertive has the effect on the other of a direct and non-destructive message by which that person would not be hurt,
4. Socio-cultural context behaviour classified as assertive is appropriate to the environment and culture in which it is demonstrated and may not necessarily be considered 'assertive' in a different socio-cultural environment.

Thus Alberti and Emmons invoke some ethical dimensions to the issue of assertiveness. They are suggesting that, used correctly, assertive behaviour is not intended to hurt the other person, should not be perceived as being hurtful and that assertive behaviour is dependent upon culture and context. They further suggest that assertive behaviour can be broken down into at least the following components:

- Eye contact The assertive person is able to maintain eye contact with another person to an appropriate degree.
- Body posture The degree of assertiveness that we use is illustrated through our posture, the way in which we stand in relation to another person and the degree to which we face the other person squarely and equally.
- Distance There seems to be a relationship between the distance we put between ourselves and another person and the degree of comfort and equality we feel with that person. If we feel overpowered by the other person's presence, we will tend to stand further away from them than we would do if we felt

equal to them. Proximity in relation to others is culturally dependent but we can soon establish the degree to which we, as individuals, tend to stand away from others or feel comfortable near to them.

- Gestures   Alberti and Emmons suggest that appropriate use of hand and arm gestures can add emphasis, openness and warmth to a message and can thus emphasize the assertive approach. Lack of appropriate hand and arm gestures can suggest lack of self-confidence and lack of spontaneity.

- Facial expression/tone of voice   It is important that the assertive person is congruent in their use of facial expression (Bandler and Grinder, 1975). Congruence is said to occur when what a person says is accompanied by an appropriate tone of voice and by appropriate facial expressions. The person who is incongruent may be perceived as unassertive. An example of this is the person who says he is angry but smiles as he says it: the result is a mixed and confusing communication.

- Fluency   A person is likely to be perceived as assertive if he is fluent and smooth in his use of his voice. This may mean that those who frequently punctuate their conversation with 'ums' and 'ers' are perceived as less than assertive.

- Timing   The assertive person is likely to be able to pay attention to his 'end' of a conversation. He will not excessively interrupt the other person, nor will he be prone to leaving long silences between utterances.

- Listening   The assertive person is likely to be a good listener. The person who listens effectively not only has more confidence in his ability to maintain a conversation but also illustrates his interest in the other person. Being assertive should not be confused with being self-centred.

- Content   Finally, it is important that what is said is appropriate to the social and cultural situation in which a conversation is taking place. Any English person who has been to America will know about the unnerving silence that is likely to descend on a conversation if he uses words such as 'fag' or 'lavatory' in certain settings! So will the person who uses slang or swear words in inappropriate situations. It is important, in being perceived as assertive, that a person learns to use appropriate words and phrases.

A paradox emerges out of all these dimensions of assertive behaviour. The assertive person also has to be genuine in his presentation of self. Now if that person is too busy noticing his behaviour and verbal performance, he is likely to feel distinctly self-conscious and contrived. It would seem that assertiveness training, like other forms of interpersonal skills training, tends to go through three stages and an understanding of those stages can help to resolve that paradox.

Stage one   The person is unaware of his behaviour and unaware of the possible changes that he may bring about in order to become more assertive.

Stage two   The person begins to appreciate the various aspects of assertive behaviour, practises them and temporarily becomes clumsy and self-conscious in their use.

Stage three   The person incorporates the new behaviours into his personal repertoire of behaviours and 'forgets' them but is perceived as more assertive. The new behaviours have become a 'natural' part of the person.

It is asserted that if behaviour change in interpersonal skills training is to become relatively permanent, the person must learn to live through the rather painful second stage of the above model. Once through it, the new skills become more effective as they are incorporated into that person's everyday presentation of self.

BECOMING ASSERTIVE

In developing assertiveness in others, the trainer is clearly going to have to be able to role model assertive behaviour herself. The starting point in this field, then, is personal development if it is required. This can be gained through attendance, initially, at an assertiveness training course and later through undertaking a 'training the trainers' course. There are an increasing number of colleges and extra mural departments of universities which offer such courses and they are also often included in the list of topics offered as evening courses.

Once the trainer has developed some competence in being assertive, the following stages need to be followed in the organization of a successful training course for others:

155

Stage one A theory input which explains the nature of assertive behaviour, including its differentiation from submissive and aggressive behaviour.

Stage two A discussion of the participants' own assessment of their assertive skills or lack of them. This assessment phase may be enhanced by volunteers role playing typical situations in which they find it difficult to be assertive.

Stage three Examples of assertive behaviour from which the participants may role-model. These may be offered in the form of short video film presentations, demonstrations by the facilitator with another facilitator, demonstrations by the facilitator with a participant in the workshop or through demonstrations offered by skilled people invited into the workshop to demonstrate assertive behaviour. The last option is perhaps the least attractive as too good a performance can often lead to group participants feeling deskilled. It is easy for the less confident person to feel 'I could never do that'. For this reason, too, it is important that the facilitator running the workshop does not present herself as being too assertive but allows some 'faults' to appear. A certain amount of lack of skill in the facilitator can be reassuring to course participants.

Stage four Selection, by participants of situations that they would like to practise in order to become more confident in being assertive. Commonly requested situations, here, may include:

- responding assertively to a colleague;
- dealing with client more assertively;
- returning faulty goods to shops or returning unsatisfactory food in a restaurant;
- not responding aggressively in a discussion;
- being able to speak in front of a group of people or deliver a short paper.

These situations can then be rehearsed using the slow role play method, described above. At each stage of the role play, the participants are encouraged to reflect on their performances and adopt assertive behaviour if they have slipped into being either aggressive or submissive. Sometimes, this means replaying the role play several times. Another learning aid, here, is the use of what may be called 'perverse role play'. Here, the various situations being played out are played out by the participants as *badly as possible*. In other words, the supposedly assertive person is anything but assertive and the 'client' behaves as badly as possible. It is often out of these perverse situations that new learning about what *could* be done occurs.

Stage five   Carrying the newly learned skills back into the 'real world'. Sometimes, the very act of having practised being assertive is enough to encourage the person to practise being assertive away from the workshop. More frequently, however, there needs to be a follow-up day or a series of follow-up days in which progress, or lack of it, is discussed and further reinforcement of effective behaviour is offered.

EFFECTS OF BEING ASSERTIVE

In this section you are invited to decide to what degree you are assertive in your relationships with others. First, consider the following areas and think about the degree to which you deal assertively (or otherwise) with other people:

1. At home
2. At work, with colleagues
3. At work, with clients or patients
4. With friends
5. In shops

Now consider the following questions:

1. Which style of confrontation describes your style best:
     a. Pussyfooting?
     b. Sledgehammer?
     c. Confronting?
2. What (if anything) stops you from being assertive:
     a. Fear of rejection?
     b. Feelings of inadequacy?
     c. Feelings that other people are more important than you?
     d. Fear of reprisal?
     e. Other feelings?
3. What do you need to do to become more assertive?
4. What is likely to happen if you become more assertive?

This last question is an important one. If you are going to become more assertive, it is likely that other people will perceive you differently for a while. If you have a tendency to be the 'pussyfooting' type, they are likely to see you as rather more pushy. If you have tended towards the 'sledgehammer' approach, they may see you as rather more subdued. Either way, other people are likely to be rather upset by your new 'presentation of self' and to want the 'old you' back. It is during this period that you need most courage and perseverance. The temptation to slip back to old ways is likely to be strong. If you want to deal with the world more on your own terms and to reduce the stress of always being subservient to the needs of others, such courage and perseverance pay off in the longer term.

SUMMARY OF THE CHAPTER

In order to care for others we must become more clear about our own needs and wants. If we want to reduce interpersonal stress we need assertiveness skills. The chapter has described the nature of assertiveness and offered a format for teaching and learning assertiveness.

REFERENCES

Alberti, R.E. and Emmons, M.L. (1982) *Your Perfect Right: a Guide to Assertive Living*, Impact, San Luis Obispo, California.

Bandler, R. and Grinder, J. (1975) *The Structure of Magic*, Vol. I, Science and Behaviour Books, California.

Hargie, O., Saunders, C. and Dickson, D. (1987) *Social Skills in Interpersonal communications*, 2nd edn, Croom Helm, London.

Heron, J. (1986) *Six Category Intervention Analysis*, 2nd Edn, Human Potential Research Project, University of Surrey, Guildford, Surrey.

Woodcock, M. and Francis, D. (1983) *The Unblocked Manager: a practical guide for self-development*, Gower, Aldershot.

Self-awareness skills

Aims of the chapter

In this chapter, the following issues and skills are discussed:

- the nature of self-awareness
- self-awareness skills
- self-presentation

WHAT IS SELF-AWARENESS?

We all need self-awareness. It is the basic prerequisite for all health care professionals. But why? This chapter lays out some of the reasons why all health care professionals need to develop self-awareness in order to enhance their care. It also explores the complicated issue of what it means to talk about 'self'.

PHILOSOPHERS AND THE SELF

What do we mean when we talk about 'the self'? Of what is the self composed? Is it part of our physical make-up? Is it something spiritual? Is it something separate to the body and, if so, what is its *relationship* to the body? Questions like these have interested philosophers and theologians for centuries. These days psychologists tackle the problem.

The existential school of philosophy discussed the issue under the heading of 'ontology', the study of being. To talk of the self, in this context, is to talk of something more than just bodily existence. It is to describe the fact of being a conscious, knowing human being. Sartre (1956) has written of 'authenticity', the state of true and honest presentation of being. The authentic person, for Sartre, is one who consistently acts in accordance with her own values, wishes and feelings, making no attempt to play act or to adopt a facade. That person also recognizes the 'being' of others and realizes that when she is with someone else, that other person is also a conscious, valuing, thinking being.

Martin Buber (1958) calls this the 'I-Thou' relationship: the meeting of two people who respect each other's humanity. He contrasts the I-Thou relationship with the I-it relationship. The person who adopts an I-it stance in relationship with another person does not recognize the other as a human being (with all that involves) but treats the other as an 'object'.

R.D. Laing wrote of the 'true' and 'false' self (Laing, 1959). The true self, according to Laing, is the inner, private sense of self. The false self is the outer, often pretending sense of self. Laing suggested that the true self often watches what the false self is doing and a sense of contempt is experienced. The false self is often compliant to the demands of others and can be artificial and insincere. In Sartre's terms, the false self acts unauthentically.

The person who has a strong sense of the true self, who is able to act authentically and genuinely is deemed by Laing to have ontological security: security and strength of being. Such security can enable the person to feel able to act rather than to feel acted upon, to make decisions and to feel generally more autonomous. Such a person is also likely to respect the autonomy and self-respect of others. This is not to be confused with selfishness or arrogance — quite the opposite. The ontologically secure person is all too aware of human frailty but, despite it, remains deter-mined to act in a genuine and honest way. It takes courage to be this way.

We can see examples of Sartre's and Laing's ideas in health care practice. When I was a patient in hospital, I became very aware of how some health care professionals adopt the 'role of the health care professional' as they enter a ward: they suddenly become 'someone else'. It is as though they leave part of them- selves behind as they go to work. They have one 'self' for their patients and another for friends and colleagues. If we notice that we are 'acting the role of the health care professional' in talking with patients, rather than being ourselves, then we are acting in an unauthentic manner.

This is not a plea for lack of professionalism but just to note that there is a world of difference between the health care professional who is open, genuine and sincere and the one who adopts a professional facade, an artificial manner and who fools no-one — neither herself, her colleagues and least of all her patients. The health care professional who begins to develop self-awareness can monitor her behaviour and note tendencies towards adopting such a veneer.

PSYCHOLOGISTS AND THE SELF

Psychologists have approached the concept of self from a variety of points of view. Some have attempted to analyse the factors that go to make up the self rather in the way that a cook might try to discover the ingredients that have gone into a cake. Others have argued that there are certain consistent aspects of the self that determine to some extent the way in which we conduct our lives.

Psychoanalytical theory, for instance, argues that early childhood experiences profoundly affect and shape the self, determining how as adults we react to the world about us. Childhood experiences, in this model, lay foundations of the self which may be modified through the process of growing up but which, nevertheless, stay with us throughout our lives. Such a view is 'deterministic': our present sense of self is determined by earlier life experiences.

Other psychologists acknowledge problems with reductionist theories — theories that attempt to analyse the self into parts. They prefer to view the self from a holistic or gestalt perspective. The gestalt approach argues that the whole or totality of the self is always something different from and larger than the sum of the aspects that make it up. Just as we cannot discover the true nature of a piece of music by examining the piece note by note, neither can we understand the self, completely, by analysing its separate aspects.

Still other psychologists take the view that the sense of self is dynamic and ever-changing. There is no core or 'real' self. What we call 'self' at any given time is that moment's set of beliefs, values and ideas that colour our view of the world. George Kelly

161

(1955) suggests the metaphor of 'goggles': we all look at the world, at ourselves and at others, through different goggles that are coloured by our beliefs, values and experiences up to that moment. As our beliefs, values and experiences change so too do the tints of our 'goggles'.

Thus, for Kelly, the person is in a constant state of flux — developing, growing and changing as she encounters life. For Kelly, we *are* what we perceive ourselves to be. Kelly also noted that we *are* what *other people* perceive us to be as well. We do not exist in isolation. What we are and who we are depends upon the other people with whom we live, work and relate. Our sense of self often depends upon the reports about us that we receive from others. In this sense, other people are telling us who we are.

As health care professionals we rely on patients, colleagues, educators and managers offering us both positive and negative feedback. We absorb such feedback and incorporate the bits that we need into our sense of self. Sometimes reports from others seem important: at other times they seem less necessary. In the exercises in Part Two of this book, this notion of receiving feedback from others is explored as part of a self-awareness programme.

ASPECTS OF THE SELF

The self, then, is a complicated concept. It is worth emphasizing the word *concept*. The self is not a *thing* in the way that our livers or lungs are 'things'. The notion of self is an abstraction, a way of talking. It is a shorthand for that part of us that is concerned with thinking, feeling, valuing, evaluating, etc. Whilst, in one sense, the mind and body are one, in another, they are different if only in that the mind is a *thing*, an object in the world, whilst the 'self' is a construct. To talk about the 'mind and body' is tricky for it is to suggest that two similar sorts of items are under discussion. One way of clarifying what is contained within the concept of self is to consider the notion of *personhood*.

If we can identify those basic criteria that distinguish persons from other sorts of things we may be clearer about what it means to talk about the self. Bannister and Fransella maintain that such a list of criteria for personhood will include at least the following items. It is argued that you consider yourself a person in that you:

1. entertain a notion of your own separateness from others: you rely on the privacy of your own consciousness;
2. entertain a notion of the integrality or completeness of your experience, so that all parts of it are relatable because you are the experiencer;
3. entertain a notion of your own continuity over time; you possess your own biography and live in relation to it;
4. entertain a notion of the causality of your actions; you have purposes, intentions, you accept a partial responsibility for the effects of what you do;
5. entertain a notion of other persons by analogy with yourself; you assume a comparability of subjective experience. (Bannister and Fransella, 1986)

These criteria bring together many of the ideas discussed above. They acknowledge the person's uniqueness and difference to others; they acknowledge the person's continuity with the past and they acknowledge her relatedness with other people. We do not exist in isolation: we can assume that we share the planet with other people who are, to a greater or lesser degree, like us.

Another way of considering the concept of self is to consider *aspects* of it. Whilst, as we have noted, all the aspects tend to work together (we hope!), in harmony, they are most easily discussed as parts. John Rowan has taken something of a similar approach in his discussion of 'subpersonalities' (Rowan, 1989) which he describes as semi-permanent, semi-autonomous regions of the personality. The analysis offered here is not an exhaustive one of all aspects of the self (as we noted above, what *individuals* call 'self' will vary from person to person). It is offered as a means of highlighting the complex and multifaceted nature of the concept of self. The aspects of self discussed here are:

1. the physical aspect
2. the spiritual aspect
3. the darker aspect
4. the social aspect
5. the private aspect

The physical aspect of self

The physical aspect of the self is the bodily, 'felt' sense of self; it includes the totality of our physical bodies. One way of considering the self, in fact, is to consider that sense as being a product of the body: bodies generate 'selves'. After all, the chemistry that goes to make up our bodies is also the chemistry that produces our 'mind', that, in turn, produces our sense of self. The physical aspect of self covers all those things such as how we feel about our bodies, our sense of body image, our appreciation of how fat or thin we are and so on. It is notable (rather painfully, some-times) that *our own* perception of our body is not necessarily the perception that others have.

The spiritual aspect of self

Human beings seem to have an inbuilt need to invest what they do with meaning. The spiritual dimension of the person may best be described as that part that is concerned with the generation of meaning. For some, that sense of meaning will be framed in religious terms but it may not be. For others, meaning may be discovered through philosophy, politics, psychology, sociology and so on. People's meaning systems vary both in their overall structure and in their content.

One thing seems certain: it is meaning (or the search for it) that motivates us for much of the time. Jung (1978) described this question for meaning as 'individuation': the search for the self which is both lonely and difficult. He suggested that one possible outcome of individuation is the realization of both the individual nature of the person and also the person's unity with all other persons. In this context, Carl Rogers noted that 'what is most personal is most general' (Rogers, 1967). There is a certain universality about the business of being human.

The darker aspect of self

There is an aspect in all of us that tends towards the negative. Whilst it has become popular to discuss the positive aspects of the self and to theorize about Maslow's (1972) notion of self-actualization — the realization of our full potential — there seems little doubt that we also have a darker side. Jung described this darker side as 'The Shadow' and wrote about it thus:

Unfortunately there is no doubt that man is, as a whole, less good than he imagines himself or wants to be. Everyone carries

a shadow, and the less it is embodied in the individual's conscious life, the blacker and denser it is . . . (Jung, 1978)

Jung suggests that if we want truly to become self-aware, we
must be prepared to explore that darker side to our personalities.
No easy task! Most of us would rather deny that side of ourselves
or rationalize our negative thoughts and behaviour. Sometimes,
however, we give ourselves away, particularly through the use of
the mental mechanism known as 'projection'. With projection we
label others with qualities that are our own but of which we are
unaware. Often we notice the bad bits of other people whilst
studiously avoiding our own. This is very evident when we
become judgemental and pious about other people. Whilst the
shadow may not be the easiest aspect of ourselves to face, it is
likely that acknowledging the darker side can help us to accept
the darker side of others.

The social aspect of self

The social self is that aspect of the person that is shared with
others. It is our presentation of self in various social situations.
Consider, for example, you at work. Consider, then, you at
home. Finally, consider you with your closest friend. You may
well find that you are considering almost three different people!
We tend to modify aspects of our presentation of self according
to the people we are with and according to what we anticipate
will be their expectations of us.

This social self, then, is closely linked to the self as defined by
others. We do not live as isolated beings. We are dependent
upon others to tell us about ourselves. More than that, we *are*
different for other people. Consider how the following people
view you: your mother, your teacher, you boy- or girlfriend. In
each case, those people will see a different 'you' and yet they are
all looking at the same person.

The private aspect of self

The private aspect of self is the part that we show only to a few
close friends, if we show it at all. It is the part of us that we are
caught up in when we are on our own. Think, for example, of the

times that you have been at home on your own. At that time, you were likely to be most completely 'yourself' — you didn't have to put up any sort of 'front' for others. As we get to know other people well, we let them glimpse little bits of the private aspect, although it is likely that we retain some aspects of the private self completely to ourselves.

These aspects of self are just that — aspects. Taken on their own, they do not convey the richness that makes us a human being. That richness is only apparent when all of the aspects are working together (and sometimes are in conflict). It is this 'gestalt' or whole that makes up the totality of self. Any attempt to break down the self into parts is bound to fail to some degree. We do not operate as 'parts' but as an integrated whole.

MODELS OF THE SELF

What is required now is a model that helps to bring all of these aspects into perspective. In its simplest form, the self as a totality can be seen as being made up of three areas or focuses of interest. These three domains are thoughts, feelings and behaviour. Each is intimately linked with the other. By thoughts is meant the processes of ideas, puzzlement, problem-solving that make up our mental life. By feelings is meant the emotional aspects of our being: happiness, grief, love, anger, joy, etc. Behaviour refers to any action that we carry out, to the spoken word and to what is usually called non-verbal behaviour: eye contact, racial expressions, gestures, proximity to others.

All three aspects of self in this simple model overlap. We cannot think without in some way feeling. Feelings lead to changes in behaviour even though these are sometimes very small changes. Try this. If someone is in the room with you now, just notice them and observe how you can tell that they are thinking or feeling. You will observe changes in eye contact, facial expression or perhaps arm or leg movements. That behaviour changes again if they notice that you are looking at them — their thinking and feeling changes as they become aware of you and their behaviour changes as a result. We cannot *stop* behaving any more than we can stop communicating.

This interrelatedness of thinking, feeling and behaviour is noticeable from any other starting point. If we ponder for a moment on how we are feeling, such pondering involves thinking

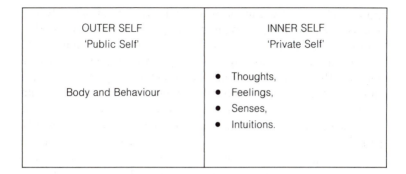

OUTER SELF 'Public Self'	INNER SELF 'Private Self'
Body and Behaviour	• Thoughts, • Feelings, • Senses, • Intuitions.

Figure 12.1   A model of the self

and, in turn, a change in behaviour. Here, then, is a starting point for approaching the study of the self. We may study each of the domains and come to know something more about ourselves. As we study each domain and appreciate the connections between all three we gradually peel back the layers to a deeper understanding of who we are. The exercises in the second half of this book will focus on all three domains.

This is a simple model of the self. A more complex model which, whilst compatible with the first, opens up the domains and expands them (Figure 12.1). It incorporates Jung's work on the four functions of the mind: thinking, feeling, sensing and intuiting (Jung, 1978) and also an adaptation of Laing's concept of the real and false self, alluded to above. It also assimilates some of the aspects of self referred to in the discussion so far.

The model is divided into two parts. The outer, public aspect of the self is what others see of us. The inner, public aspect is what goes on in our heads and bodies. In one way, the outer experience is what other people are most familiar with. We communicate the inner experience through the outer. Our thoughts and feelings are all communicated through this outer presentation of self. Of what does it consist?

THE OUTER EXPERIENCE OF THE SELF

At the most obvious, behaviour consists of body movements: the turning of the head, the crossing of arms and legs, walking and running and so on. At a more subtle level the issue becomes more involved. We can note a whole variety of less obvious behaviours that convey something about the inner sense of self.

First is speech. Clearly what we say, the words and phrases we use, are a potent means by which we convey thoughts and feelings to others. How we come to choose *these* particular words and phrases, however, depends on our past experiences, our education, our social position, our attitudes, values and beliefs and on the company that we are in when we use those words. Running alongside speech are the non-linguistic aspects of speech: timing, pacing, volume, minimal prompts ('mm's and 'yes's), the use of silence, etc. The use of such non-linguistic aspects of speech can be a powerful way of conveying our inner selves to others. As we noted above, we are always communicating, even when we think we are not!

When we talk to others we invariably look at them. As Heron (1970) notes there can be a wide variety in the intensity, amount and quality of eye contact. When we are embarrassed or upset, for example, we make less eye contact. When we are emotionally close to another person, our eye contact is often sustained. We can learn to become conscious of our use of what must be the most powerful aspect of communication and to monitor the amount and quality of our eye contact. We should also remain aware of the *cultural* differences that are involved here. People from cultures very different from our own use eye contact in other ways. It is important that we do not interpret such different use of eye contact inappropriately.

Touch is another important aspect of our outer experience. Typically, in this culture, we touch more those people to whom we are close: members of the family, lovers and very close friends. Health care involves a high degree of this personal aspect of human interaction and it is important that, as with eye contact, we learn to monitor and consciously use the facility of touch. It is worth noting, too, that some people are 'high touchers' and others 'low touchers'. Some people like being touched and like touching others; other people are repelled by it. Also, all touching should be unambiguous — clearly touch has sexual connotations for some people.

When we communicate verbally with others, we tend to stand or sit close to them. How near we stand or sit in relation to others is determined by a number of factors: the level of intimacy we have with them, our relationship with them and whether or not we are dominant or submissive in that relationship (Brown,

1965). In the health care professions, people tend to be in a dominant position *vis-à-vis* their patients and clients and tend to stand closer to those patients and clients than would be the case in ordinary day-to-day relationships.

It is useful to imagine that we are surrounded by an invisible bubble, the threshold of which can only be crossed by certain other people. If people accidentally break through the bubble and touch us, they tend to withdraw quickly to avoid embarrassment to both parties. The issue of proximity to others needs close consideration. We need to become aware of how close or distant we like to be to others. We also need to note other people's preferences and to be sensitive towards them. One useful way of judging this distance between you and the other person is to allow the other person to set that distance. In other words, you invite the other person to draw up a chair or you allow them to determine where they will stand in relation to you and not vice versa. Once again, as we become more self-aware, so we gain more insight into the needs and wants of others.

One of the clearest indicators of our inner experience is facial expression. Frowns and smiles do much to convey the feelings that are being experienced inside. It is important that facial expression and speech are congruent or matched. We have all experienced the person who says that they are cheerful or upset but whose facial expression suggests otherwise. Bandler and Grinder (1975) note that for the purposes of clear communication, three aspects of our outer behaviour must match: general body position, content of speech and facial expression. If two or more of these are mismatched then our communication will be confused and confusing. Thus if we say that we are cheerful but shrug our shoulders and have an unhappy expression, the message will be unclear. We can do a lot to improve our communication on this level. It is insufficient just to *say* what we mean. We must be *seen* to mean it as well.

Two issues become clear from this brief analysis of the outer aspects of self. We can become aware of our use of speech, eye contact, touch, proximity to others, gesture, facial expression and non-linguistic aspects of speech as a means of deepening our understanding of ourselves. Also, by becoming conscious of how we use those verbal and non-verbal behaviours we can use them more skilfully to enhance our contact with others. We can increase our interpersonal skills by intentionally using ourselves as instruments. Heron uses the expression 'conscious use of self'

(Heron, 1977) to convey this concept. This is not to say that we need to become robotic and artificial but to note that in caring for others we can more precisely use our 'selves' as instruments of communication.

THE INNER EXPERIENCE

The inner, private experience in this model may be divided into four aspects of mental functioning — thinking, feeling, sensing and intuition — and the experience of the body. Clearly, the division of these aspects into two groups is artificial as both mental and physical events are interrelated. As Searle (1983) points out, a mental event is also a physical event. To think that it is not to perpetuate the old philosophical problem of mind/ body dualism. This is sometimes known as Cartesian dualism after the philosopher René Descartes, who believed that mental and physical events could be considered separately. Today, the tendency is towards healing this split and interest continues to develop in concepts of holistic medicine — which treat the mind and body together. As we have already noted, any concept of the self must take into account the mind and the body as a totality.

The thinking dimension

In this model, thinking refers to all the aspects, logical and otherwise, of our mental processes. One moment's reflection on thinking will reveal that it is not a linear process. We do not think in sentences or even in a series of phrases. The process is much more haphazard than that. The technique known as 'free-association' and used in psychoanalysis demonstrates the apparently random nature of some of our thinking. Free association demands the individual verbalizes whatever comes into her mind, without any attempt at censoring or stopping the flow. Try to do this. The process is always difficult and sometimes impossible. The reasons for this are outlined in the psychoanalytical literature and such theory can offer insights into the genesis and nature of thought processes. Clearly, not everybody wants or can afford psychoanalysis but its ideas can be useful in attempting to understand thinking.

Arguably, the domain of thinking is more dominant in certain individuals. Certainly, thinking is highly rated in our culture and the education system sometimes seems to concern itself only with this. The domains of feeling, sensing and intuiting are usually less well catered for. In the health professions, however, we are concerned with all sorts of feelings, from pain to anxiety, from depression to elation. Understanding these requires the use of dimensions other than thinking. On the other hand, it is obviously important that we all develop thinking. If we are to progress as a research-based profession and if we are to be able to demonstrate critical awareness, we must be able to think clearly. We must also be able to appreciate when feeling gets in the way of thinking, and vice versa.

The feeling dimension

Feeling in this model refers to the emotional aspect of the person: love, sadness, joy, happiness, etc. Heron (1977) argues that there are four dominant aspects of emotion that are frequently denied and repressed in our culture: anger, grief, fear and embarrassment. He argues that anger can be expressed through loud sound and shouting, grief through tears, fear through trembling and embarrassment through laughter. He argues further that such expression of emotion (or catharsis) is a healthy process. Heron claims that we live in a non-cathartic culture and the general tendency is to encourage people to control rather than to express emotion. As a result, we all carry round with us a pool of unexpressed emotion which distorts our thinking and stops us functioning fully. If we can learn to express some of this bottled up emotion and methods of doing this will be discussed later, then we can become more open to experience, less fearful and anxious and we can exercise more self-determination and autonomy. Part of becoming self-aware entails discovering and exploring the emotional dimension.

Health care professionals must deal with other people's emotions and there is a positive link between the way in which we handle our own emotions and the way in which we handle those of others. If we understand and can appropriately express our own anger, fear, grief and embarrassment, we will be better able to handle them in other people. In caring for others, we must get to know ourselves better.

Certainly other people's emotions affect us and stir up our

own, unexpressed emotions. Try this simple experiment. Next time a programme on television moves you near to tears, turn off the set and allow yourself to cry. As you do so, reflect on what it is you are crying about. It is highly likely that the issue causing the tears is a personal one, not directly related to the tele- vision programme. Most people carry around with them this unexpressed emotion, just beneath the surface. Health care professionals who work in particularly emotionally charged environments — children's wards, intensive therapy units, psychi- atric units, etc. — may want to consider self-help methods for exploring their own hidden emotions. Co-counselling, discussed in the next chapter, is one such method and others are discussed by Bond (1986) and Bond and Kilty (1982). Alternatively, con- sider going to the cimema as a means of emotional release. What do most people go to the cinema for? To cry, to allow them- selves to become frightened or to laugh. The cinema, the theatre, concerts and sporting events offer 'natural' release valves for people's pent-up emotions.

The sensing dimension

The sensing dimension in the model refers to inputs through the five special senses, touch, taste, smell, hearing, sight, and also to proprioceptive and kinaesthetic sense. Proprioception refers to our ability to know the position of our bodies and thus to know where we are in space. We do not, for instance, need to *think* about our body position most of the time. We are fed that information by bundles of nerve fibres known as proprioceptors. Kinaesthetic sense refers to our sense of body movement. Again, this is not a sense that we normally have to think about.

We can make ourselves aware of any of the senses. Another simple experiment will demonstrate this. Stop reading for a moment and pay attention to everything that you can hear. Take in all the sounds around you: the more subtle as well as the more obvious. In doing so, notice how much of this one particular sense is normally passed over and how many sounds are usually filtered out of consciousness. At times it is vital that our senses are selective and that extraneous sounds, images, smells and so on are banished from awareness. On the other hand, often that filtering mechanism becomes too efficient and we filter out or fail to notice many sounds and sights that are around us all the time. We live half asleep.

In developing an awareness of our senses, we can begin to notice the world again. Just as importantly, we can begin to notice each other again. In developing our sense of sight, for instance, we can begin to notice subtle changes in other people's expressions, body postures and other aspects of non-verbal communication. Without that awareness we may miss a considerable amount of essential interpersonal information. In health care, the value of such awareness is clear. Health care professionals need to be observant. What is not always so clear is *how* health care professionals are supposed to become observant. Like any other skills development, training to notice takes time and practice. The redeeming feature is that it is a skill which the *individual* can develop for herself. In a way, it is simply a matter of *remembering* to notice. Eventually, such awareness or 'staying awake' becomes part of the person.

The intuitive dimension

The intuitive dimension is perhaps the most undervalued. Intuition refers to the knowledge and insight that arrives independently of the senses. In other words we just 'know'. Ornstein (1975) who studies the literature on the differences between the two sides of the brain identified intuition with the right side. He argued that the two sides have qualitatively different functions. The left side is concerned with cognitive processes and with rationality. The right is more to do with holism, creativity and intuition, according to Ornstein. If he is right, the implication is that if the intuitive aspect is developed further (along with creativity) then both sides of the brain will function optimally. Ornstein argues that the present Western culture is dominated by the left brain approach to education and development. He calls for an educational system that honours creativity and intuition alongside the development of rationality.

Perhaps we neglect intuition through fear of it or concern that it may not be trusted. On the other hand, it is likely that we all have 'hunches' that when followed turn out to be 'right'. Many aspects of health care require the health care professional to be intuitive. Sometimes, in order to empathize with another person we have to guess at what they are feeling. Sometimes we seem to

173

'know' what they are feeling. Certainly, group work and counselling depend to a fair degree on this intuitive ability. Carl Rogers, founder of client-centred counselling, noted that when he had a hunch about something that was happening in a counselling session, it invariably helped if he verbalized that intuition (Rogers, 1967). Using intuition consciously and openly takes courage and sometimes it is wrong. One the other hand, used hand in hand with more traditional forms of thinking, it can enhance the health care professional/patient relationship in a way that logic on its own never can.

The experience of the body

The third aspect of the model of self-awareness is the experience of the body. If the mind and body are directly interrelated, in fact inseparable, then any mental activity will affect the body, and vice versa.

It is easy to talk as though the mind and body are separate. Indeed we do not *have* a mind/body, we *are* our mind/body. Everything that we refer to as being part of our mind and body is part of our selves. Expressions such as 'I'm not happy with my body . . . ' or 'I've got that sort of mind . . .' indicate how easy it is for us to dissociate ourselves from either the body or the mind.

Coming to notice body feelings takes time and patience. Of course, appreciation of inner bodily experiences are limited to some degree by the supply of sensory nerve endings to certain parts of the body. Some are better served than others. On the other hand it is easy to lose touch with those bodily sensations of which we *may* become aware. Before you read any further, just take a moment to notice what is going on inside your body. What do you notice? Are there areas of muscle tension? Are the muscles of your stomach pulled in tightly? Can you become aware of your breathing? Are you breathing deeply into your stomach or is your breathing light and shallow? What happens when you make small changes to your body? What happens when you relax sets of muscles or change your breathing?

All of the information that can be gleaned from the body can enable us to appreciate something about our psychological status. Tension in sets of muscles, for example, may be the first we know of the fact that we are anxious or tense. Learning to 'listen' to the body in this way can help us more accurately to assess our true feelings about ourselves and others.

Wilhelm Reich (1949), a psychoanalyst who was particularly interested in the mind/body relationship, advanced the notion of 'character armour'. Reich maintained that our emotional feelings could become trapped within sets of muscles and consequently affected posture and movement. He suggested that direct manipulation of those sets of muscles could release the emotion trapped within them with characteristic emotional release of catharsis. Such work on the body has become known as Reichian bodywork and can be a powerful and effective means of developing self-awareness through direct body contact.

Similar but different methods of this sort which involve direct physical contact include Rolfing (Rolf, 1973), bioenergetics (Lowen, 1967) and Feldenkrais (Feldenkrais, 1972), three body-work methods that have developed out of Reich's original formulation. Less dramatic but valid methods of body/mind exploration include massage, yoga, the martial arts, certain types of meditation, the Alexander technique (Alexander, 1969), dance and certain types of sport.

All these methods can enhance awareness of self through attention to changes in the body and thus create insight into psychological states. They can also aid the development of awareness of body image. Observations of people in everyday life will reveal how frequently people walk around with lop-sided shoulders, a stooping gait or even with either side of their face showing different expressions. Often, too, they seem to be totally unaware of these things. Bodywork methods can enable the individual to develop greater physical symmetry and balance, better posture, improved breathing and a healthier physical status, generally. All aspects of health care call for psychological and physical stamina and are taxing on the mind/body. These methods in combination with more traditional approaches to self-awareness can lead to a powerful and healthy approach to self-care. Perhaps burnout, so frequently a problem of occupations that depend upon a high degree of human contact, can be prevented effectively through this mix of attention to the body and mind.

SELF-AWARENESS

A model of the self has been outlined which takes account of the inner and outer aspects of the concept and which has attempted to marry the mind and body. The question now arises: what is self-awareness?

A first point that needs to be made is that what is *not* being discussed is 'self-consciousness', in the everyday sense of the word. To be self-conscious is to be embarrassed by ourselves, to be painfully aware of our being observed by others. Sartre (1956) describes this well when he suggests that under the scrutinizing gaze of the other person, we are turned into an object, a 'thing'. It is our response to being treated in this way that causes us to become self-conscious. For the very self-conscious person, this sense of being treated as an object is exaggerated by that person herself. In being too acutely aware of other people's attention, she imagines herself to be more acutely scrutinized than is actually the case. It is rather like having someone watch us undertaking a skill such as giving an injection. We tend a) to become deskilled by their watching us and b) imagine that they are being highly critical. Self-consciousness is a bit like this. It tends to make you awkward and tends to make you feel criticized. This is true, for example, of the adolescent who imagines (usually falsely) that they are being looked at with highly critical eyes. Their own sense of insecurity is projected onto the world and they imagine that others view them as harshly and as critically as they view themselves.

Clearly, such self-consciousness is more of a hindrance than a help when it comes to relating to others, as any acutely shy person knows. Yet such self-consciousness is far removed from self-awareness and may indicate a false or exaggerated self-concept.

Self-awareness refers to the gradual and continuous process of noticing and exploring aspects of the self, whether behavioural, psychological or physical, with the intention of developing personal and interpersonal understanding. Such awareness is probably best not developed for its own sake: it is intimately bound up with our relationships with others. To become more aware of and to have a deeper understanding of ourselves is to have a sharper and clearer picture of what is happening to others.

In this sense, it is a process of discrimination. The more that we can discriminate ourselves from others, the more we can understand our similarities. If we are unaware and blind to our own selves then we are likely to remain blind to others. A rather crude illustration may help to drive this point home. If I buy a red sweater, I immediately notice how many other people are wearing red sweaters — a fact of which I was not aware before the purchase. In noticing that fact about others I can also notice other things about them. And so, if I let it, the process escalates. I can notice more subtle differences between persons but also their similarities. The point is that the process begins with me. I must first examine myself.

Such a process of examination requires patience and honesty. It is easy to fall into the trap of interpreting thoughts, feelings and behaviour, rather than (initially at least) merely noticing them. That interpretation logically comes *after* we have gathered the data, after we have clearly described to ourselves our present status. This stage of self-awareness training may be likened to the assessment stage of the diagnosis process. Information about the self is gathered in order to develop a clearer picture, before any attempt is made to solve problems, decide upon changes, or identify reasons for the way we are.

This approach may be described as a phenomenological one (Spinelli, 1989). Phenomenology is a branch of philosophy that is concerned with attempting to describe things as they appear to be without recourse to making value-judgements about them. Thus, in the human context, a phenomenological approach to self-awareness training would concern itself purely with describing aspects of the self as they surface and become known. Such an approach demands that we suspend judgement on ourselves. Instead of telling ourselves that 'this bit of me is O.K . . . this bit is bad and needs to be changed', we merely note that it *is as it is*. Once we have more data at our disposal, the answer to the question 'why?' may become self-evident. To jump to hasty conclusions may be either a) to be harshly critical of ourselves or b) to wreck the project altogether because we are disenchanted. Certainly, the road to self-awareness is not an easy one to tread, but the phenomenological approach can make it bearable. After all, if *we* don't accept ourselves, who will? If we don't accept ourselves, will we accept other people?

This method of description rather than interpretation is of great value in group settings and in counselling. When experiential learning is discussed in the next chapter, the notion of the phenomenological role of the facilitator is described. In this role, the facilitator of the group does not attempt to offer interpretations of what is happening in the group but limits herself to descriptions of events and of behaviours and encourages other group members to do the same. In the context of counselling, the phenomenological approach also pays dividends. If we can stand back and avoid interpreting what it is we think our clients are saying, we give them the chance to make their own interpreta-tions. This attitude towards counselling is known as the client-centred approach (Rogers, 1967; Burnard, 1989). It is argued that the only person who *can* make a valid interpretation of her behaviour is the person herself.

DEVELOPING SELF-AWARENESS

There are various ways of developing self-awareness. Some involve introspection and others entail involvement with and feedback from other people. Any course leading towards self-awareness must contain both facets: the inner search and the observations of others. Introspection by itself can lead to a one-sided, totally subjective view of the self. It is difficult, if not impossible, for the person working on her own to transcend herself and take the larger view. In order to balance that subjec-tive view, we need the view of others.

Before examining some of the methods of introspection and group work, it is useful to note one simple method of enhancing self-awareness: the process of noticing what we are doing, the process of self-monitoring. All that is involved here is that you stay conscious of what you are doing, as you do it. In other words, you 'stay awake' and develop the skill of keeping your attention focused on your actions, both verbal and non-verbal. Such a process, whilst easy in theory, can in practice be quite difficult. It is easy to become distracted by inner thoughts and preoccupations so that our actions become automatic and unnoticed — even robotic.

All such explorations can be carried out either in isolation, with another person or in groups. To explore the self in the company of another person can be a rewarding and economical method. Economical in that the time available can be equally divided between the two people. Co-counselling offers a useful format for such exploration. This is a process by which two people who are trained as co-counsellors meet and spend equal time in the role of counsellor and client. Co-counselling is a self-awareness method which is taught by various trainers in colleges and extra-mural departments of universities.

Other methods of self-awareness training include the use of role play, social skills training, meditation and assertiveness skills training. These methods are well documented in the literature

(Kagan, 1985; Bond, 1986; Hargie, Saunders and Dickson, 1987; Burnard, 1989) and courses in these forms of training are frequently organized by women's groups, growth centres and extramural departments of colleges and universities.

In health care professional education and training, the use of videos can enhance self-awareness by allowing students to view themselves as if from another person's point of view. Such training, however, should always be voluntary. Some people find the use of video taping a gross invasion of personal territory and the method should be used with discretion.

As we have noted, work on the body via Reichian body work, yoga, tai chi, the martial arts and sport all have their place in self-awareness development both for their effects on the body but also for their limit-testing capacity. A quieter, more reflective approach is the use of journals or diaries and these can be used to monitor self-awareness development alongside educational development.

Probably the ideal is a combination of a variety of approaches: introspection, with a group, active and passive. In this way, the self is studied in all its aspects and in a variety of contexts. As we have noted, the 'self' is not a static once-and-for-all thing but an entity that is constantly changing depending, amongst other things, on the people we are with. The eclectic approach is also healthier in that it encourages the combination of sport and exercise alongside meditation and more reflective practices. It also allows for normal social relationships to develop alongside periods of solidarity. No-one ever became self-aware by shutting themselves away from the rest of the world. Also, it is important that self-awareness development has a practical end — the enhancement of interpersonal relationships and skills.

SELF-AWARENESS AND THE HEALTH CARE PROFESSIONALS

Having explored the concept of self and examined some methods of self-awareness development, the question remains: why develop self-awareness anyway?

In the first instance, to discover more about ourselves is to differentiate ourselves from others. If we cannot differentiate between our own thoughts and feelings and those of others, we stand to blur our ego boundaries, our sense of ourself as an independent, autonomous being. Conversely, if we constantly blur the distinction between 'you and me', we risk not recognizing the other person's independence and autonomy. When ego boundaries are blurred, we lose the sense of whose problem is whose. With self-awareness we can learn to distinguish between our problems and those of others, and vice versa. This is particularly important in sensitive areas such as psychiatry and care of the dying person. Real involvement and care in these fields also involves (almost paradoxically) the ability to detach ourselves a little in order to get things into perspective. If we cannot engage in this distancing we risk being drawn into other people's problems to such a degree that we can no longer help them. Their problems have become ours.

To become self-aware is also to learn conscious use of the self. We become agents: we are able to choose to act rather than feeling acted upon. We learn to select therapeutic interventions from a range of options so that the patient or client benefits more completely. If we are blind to ourselves we are also blind to our choices. We are blind, then, to caring and therapeutic choices that we could make on behalf of our patients.

Once we can combine two aspects — differentiation from others and an increased awareness of the range of therapeutic choices available to use — we can be more sensitive to the needs and wants of others. We can even choose to *forget ourselves* in order to give ourselves more completely to others. No longer do we run the risk of being sucked into other people's problems, nor do we confuse our thoughts and feelings with those of our patients. We can offer therapeutic distance with therapeutic choice.

Interpersonal interventions such as counselling and group facilitation require that we exercise some self-awareness. All that has been discussed in the above paragraphs is particularly true when we are trying to help people in these particular sorts of therapeutic situations. In Part Two of this book, both counselling skills and group facilitation skills are explored. It is a vital prerequisite that alongside the development of such skills, the person taking part in the activities in this section will also continue to develop self-awareness. Skills development without self-awareness tends to encourage the development of a stilted and unnatural presentation of self. Without self-awareness, the person appears merely to have a set of skills 'tacked on' to her;

these skills are used neither sensitively nor awarely but in a robotic and automatic way.

PROBLEMS IN SELF-AWARENESS DEVELOPMENT

It is worth repeating the point made at various stages throughout this chapter: that the aim of self-awareness development is to enable us to increase our interpersonal skills. The path to such awareness is, however, fraught with problems. First is the problem of egocentricity. It is possible to become caught up in the idea of understanding the self to the degree that it becomes an end in itself. This tends to lead to the person becoming self-indulgent and self-centred. Clearly such positions are not compatible with altruism or concern for others. Second, it is possible for those who develop self-awareness to believe that they have discovered insights that set them apart or even make them better than other people. A sign of such development is sometimes the loss of a sense of humour. Life becomes very earnest.

True self-awareness, however, tends to lead to a lightness of touch and a sense of humility at the sheer scale of the task in hand. To continue with that task, it is important that the person maintains (and exercises) a sense of humour in order to keep sight of the 'larger canvas'. Certainly the best run self-awareness groups are those that offer a 'light' atmosphere. If the atmosphere becomes too heavy and earnest, it is likely to put everyone off. It is certainly not conducive to easy and frank self-disclosure.

Linked to this is the problem of the self-awareness group facilitator becoming something of a 'guru' figure. As people find things out about themselves, they sometimes tend to imagine that the group facilitator has special qualities that enable her to allow this to happen. As a result, those people tend to set the facilitator up as some sort of heroine. Sometimes, too, the facilitator believes in this image and ends up acting out the role of guru.

Again, caution and humility are keywords. Both group members and facilitator should remember that the facilitator is human, like everyone else. I use the word 'she', here, but in my experience (and for whatever reason) it is nearly always men who either set themselves up in the guru role or are put in it by their groups.

Finally comes the issue of voluntariness. Self-awareness cannot be forced upon people. Facilitators of self-awareness groups would do well to exercise what Heron (1977) calls the voluntary principle. This is a principle invoked at the beginning of any self-awareness training course and repeated at intervals throughout such a course that no-one at any time will have pressure exerted on them to take part and that everyone takes part in any exercise of their own free will. If self-awareness is about developing autonomy and the exercise of choice, it is important that such autonomy and choice begins with deciding whether or not a given exercise suits them at this time. Accepting and respecting other people's frailties, their reserve and their choice not to disclose aspects of themselves until they are ready are all part of the process of facilitation. Such understanding on the part of the facilitator will do much to increase the confidence of group members and to create an atmosphere conducive to self-understanding.

PRESENTATION OF SELF

You are an instrument of communication. What you wear, what you say, the way that you say it: all of these communicate who you are to others. We have at least two choices. One is not to take any notice of the how and the what of personal communication. The other is to choose how we communicate. Heron (1977) refers to this as 'conscious use of the self'. In the following paragraphs you are invited to reflect on aspects of self-presentation. During the process, try to make decisions about what and how you need to change (if at all). If you are someone who frequently thinks about their presentation of self, the activity will not be too difficult. If you are someone who infrequently thinks about who and what you are, then the process may be less easy.

PRESENTATION OF SELF QUESTIONNAIRE

Work through the following questions and think about the way you present yourself to others.

Clothes

- Do you have different sorts of clothes for work and for home?
- If so, how do you make decisions about what sorts of clothes to buy for each situation?

- Do you consciously strive for a particular style?
- What sort of style is it?
- When did you last change the style?
- Why do you adopt it?

Introductions

- How do you introduce yourself to others?
- How do you introduce yourself on the telephone?
- How do you introduce other people to friends and colleagues?
- Is it something you find easy or difficult?
- How could you improve your introductions?

Holding a conversation

- Are you a good listener?
- What do you do while you listen?
- Are you a 'sentence finisher' when others are talking?
- Do you think you talk too much?
- Are you shy in conversations?
- To what degree do you self-disclose?
- How do you handle other people's self-disclosure?
- What do you do when you find yourself becoming emotional in a conversation?
- What are you like at handling other people's emotions?

Ending conversations

- What do you do when you want to finish a conversation?
- How do you finish a phone conversation?
- Do you find that people keep on talking to you even though you think you have indicated that you have to stop?
- What do you need to do to improve the way that you finish a conversation?

Non-verbal communication

- Do you look at people when you talk to them?
- Are you comfortable making eye contact with other people?
- In what situations are you *not* comfortable making eye contact?
- What do you do with your hands when you talk?
- How do you *stand*: are you upright, slightly slouched, uncomfortable?
- What position do you adopt when you are sitting down: do you cross your legs, fold your arms?
- Do you smile very much?
- Do you tend to frown?
- How close or distant do you sit or stand in relation to other people?
- Have you ever felt uncomfortable in relation to personal space?
- Do you ever touch the other person when you speak?
- Would you say that you were a 'high toucher' or a 'low toucher'?

Content of conversations

- Is conversation a serious business to you?
- Do you gossip?
- Do you prefer light or heavy conversations?
- Is a sense of humour important to you?
- Do you talk about yourself a lot?
- Do you allow others to talk about themselves?
- Which do you prefer: talking or listening?

Your values

- What things are most important to you?
- Why are they?
- In what ways do your values affect your behaviour and the way that you live?

- Do you respect people with values different from your own?
- How do you handle conflict over values?
- Do you ever act against your values?

SUMMARY OF THE CHAPTER

We all need to become self-aware in order to offer all we can to our clients, patients and colleagues. This final chapter has discussed some ways of developing self-awareness. Just as the book opened with a universally applicable topic — learning — so the book closes with the topic that can help us all to become better communicators. In the end, all of our communication focuses round the person that we are.

REFERENCES

Alexander, F.M. (1969) *Resurrection of the Body*, University Books, New York.
Bandler, R. and Grinder, J. (1975) *The Structure of Magic*, Vol. I, Science and Behaviour Books, California.
Bannister, D. and Fransella, F. (1986) *Inquiring Man*, 3rd edn, Croom Helm, London.
Bond, M. (1986) *Stress and Self-Awareness*, Heinemann, London.
Bond, M. and Kilty, J. (1982) *Practical Methods of Coping With Stress*, Human Potential Research Project, University of Surrey, Guildford, Surrey.
Brown, R. (1965) *Social Psychology*, Collier Macmillan, London.
Buber, M. (1958) *I and Thou*, Scribner, New York.
Burnard, P. (1989) *Teaching Interpersonal Skills: A handbook of experiential learning for health professionals*, Chapman and Hall, London.
Feldenkrais, M. (1972) *Awareness Through Movement*, Harper and Row, London.
Hargie, O, Saunders, C. and Dickson, D. (1987) *Social Skills in Interpersonal Communication*, 2nd edn, Croom Helm, London.
Heron, J. (1970) *The Phenomenology of the Gaze*, Human Potential Research Project, University of Surrey, Guildford, Surrey.
Heron, J. (1977) *Behaviour Analysis in Education and Training*, Human Potential Research Project, University of Surrey, Guildford, Surrey.
Jung, C.G. (1978) *Selected Writing*, Fontana, London.
Kagan, C. (ed.) (1985) *Interpersonal Skills in Nursing*, Croom Helm, London.
Kelly, G. (1955) *The Psychology of Personal Constructs*, 2 vols, Norton, New York.

Laing, R.D. (1959) *The Divided Self*, Penguin Harmondsworth.

Lowen, A. (1967) *Betrayal of the Body*, Macmillan, New York.

Maslow, A. (1972) *Motivation and Personality*, Harper and Row, London.

Ornstein, R.E. (1975) *The Psychology of Consciousness*, Penguin, Harmondsworth.

Reich, W. (1949) *Character Analysis*, Simon and Schuster, New York.

Rogers, C.R. (1967) *On Becoming a Person*, Constable, London.

Rolf, I. (1973) *Structured Integration*, Viking Press, New York.

Rowan, J. (1989) The self: One or many? *The Psychologist, Bulletin of the British Psychological Society*, **7**, 279–81.

Sartre, J.-P. (1956) *Being and Nothingness*, Philosophical Library, New York.

Searle, J. (1983) *Philosophy of Mind*, Cambridge University Press, Cambridge.

Spinelli, J. (1989) *The Interpreted World*, Routledge, London.

Skills check: Part Four

Sit quietly and reflect on the skills that have been discussed in this section. How many of them are applicable in your health care setting? To what degree do you feel that you have had training in those that are applicable?

Now ask yourself the following questions:

- To what degree is my writing effective?
- Do I enjoy writing?
- How could I improve it?
- Am I generally assertive?
- In what situations am I not assertive?
- To what degree am I self-aware?

13

Personal communication skills questionnaire

You can use this questionnaire in various ways:

- As a self-assessment and self-evaluation instrument before, during and after reading this book;
- As a means of identifying which skills you need to work on further;
- As a basis for discussion in group work.

Read through each of the sections and ring the appropriate statement following each statement. The statements are:

Strongly agree Agree Don't know Disagree Strongly disagree

CHAPTER 1: TEACHING SKILLS

1. I am quite good at learning from my own experience
   Strongly agree Agree Don't know Disagree Strongly disagree

2. I am good at helping others to learn from their own experience
   Strongly agree Agree Don't know Disagree Strongly disagree

3. I am better at teaching than facilitating
   Strongly agree Agree Don't know Disagree Strongly disagree

4. I prefer facilitation to teaching
   Strongly agree Agree Don't know Disagree Strongly disagree

5. Most of the educational experiences I have had have been formal ones
   Strongly agree Agree Don't know Disagree Strongly disagree

6. Most health professional training is teacher-centred
   Strongly agree Agree Don't know Disagree Strongly disagree

7. Therapy is a form of education
   Strongly agree Agree Don't know Disagree Strongly disagree

CHAPTER 2: PRESENTATION SKILLS

8. The idea of making a presentation to a group of colleagues is not a daunting one
   Strongly agree Agree Don't know Disagree Strongly disagree

9. The idea of making a presentation at a conference worries me
   Strongly agree Agree Don't know Disagree Strongly disagree

10. I would handle a formal presentation better than an informal one
    Strongly agree Agree Don't know Disagree Strongly disagree

11. I would not be sure of my ability to produce effective visual aids
    Strongly agree Agree Don't know Disagree Strongly disagree

CHAPTER 3: COMPUTING SKILLS

12. I am computer literate
    Strongly agree Agree Don't know Disagree Strongly disagree

13. I do not know how to use a computer
    Strongly agree Agree Don't know Disagree Strongly disagree

189

14. I am happy with a wordprocessor but not with a spreadsheet
Strongly agree Agree Don't know Disagree Strongly disagree

15. I have no use for a computer
Strongly agree Agree Don't know Disagree Strongly disagree

CHAPTER 4: LISTENING SKILLS

16. I am not a naturally good listener
Strongly agree Agree Don't know Disagree Strongly disagree

17. I listen to other people very well
Strongly agree Agree Don't know Disagree Strongly disagree

18. I enjoy listening to others
Strongly agree Agree Don't know Disagree Strongly disagree

19. I listen to clients well, but not so well to colleagues
Strongly agree Agree Don't know Disagree Strongly disagree

CHAPTER 5: COUNSELLING SKILLS

20. I would like to be more effective as a counsellor
Strongly agree Agree Don't know Disagree Strongly disagree

21. I think counselling is part of every health professional's role
Strongly agree Agree Don't know Disagree Strongly disagree

22. I think counselling should be left to professionals
Strongly agree Agree Don't know Disagree Strongly disagree

23. I would like to learn the basics of counselling
Strongly agree Agree Don't know Disagree Strongly disagree

CHAPTER 6: GROUP SKILLS

24. I don't enjoy the prospect of running a group
Strongly agree Agree Don't know Disagree Strongly disagree

25. I enjoy being a group participant
Strongly agree Agree Don't know Disagree Strongly disagree

26. I think I would be quite effective as a small group facilitator
Strongly agree Agree Don't know Disagree Strongly disagree

27. I enjoy running groups
Strongly agree Agree Don't know Disagree Strongly disagree

CHAPTER 7: MANAGEMENT SKILLS

28. I manage people well
Strongly agree Agree Don't know Disagree Strongly disagree

29. I am fairly organized in my work
Strongly agree Agree Don't know Disagree Strongly disagree

30. I manage time effectively
Strongly agree Agree Don't know Disagree Strongly disagree

31. I would like to be better at managing people
Strongly agree Agree Don't know Disagree Strongly disagree

32. I would prefer to handle my time more effectively
Strongly agree Agree Don't know Disagree Strongly disagree

CHAPTER 8: MEETING SKILLS

33. I enjoy going to meetings
Strongly agree Agree Don't know Disagree Strongly disagree

34. I am quite effective as a chairperson
Strongly agree Agree Don't know Disagree Strongly disagree

35. I dread being asked to take the minutes
Strongly agree Agree Don't know Disagree Strongly disagree

36. Meetings are not really my cup of tea
Strongly agree Agree Don't know Disagree Strongly disagree

37. I think our organization has too many meetings
Strongly agree Agree Don't know Disagree Strongly disagree

CHAPTER 9: INTERVIEW SKILLS

38. I always get nervous if I am asked to conduct interviews
Strongly agree Agree Don't know Disagree Strongly disagree

39. I would prefer to be interviewed than to interview others
Strongly agree Agree Don't know Disagree Strongly disagree

40. I am not very organized when I interview people
Strongly agree Agree Don't know Disagree Strongly disagree

41. I am not sure how to draw up a curriculum vitae
Strongly agree Agree Don't know Disagree Strongly disagree

CHAPTER 10: WRITING SKILLS

42. I could never write anything for publication
Strongly agree Agree Don't know Disagree Strongly disagree

43. I would like to see something I had written in print
Strongly agree Agree Don't know Disagree Strongly disagree

44. I could never write a book
Strongly agree Agree Don't know Disagree Strongly disagree

45. I read a lot: perhaps I could write
Strongly agree Agree Don't know Disagree Strongly disagree

46. I have always wanted to write
Strongly agree Agree Don't know Disagree Strongly disagree

CHAPTER 11: ASSERTIVENESS SKILLS

47. I don't seem to be able to say 'no' to people very easily
Strongly agree Agree Don't know Disagree Strongly disagree

48. I would prefer to be more assertive
   Strongly agree Agree Don't know Disagree Strongly disagree

49. I think that people who say they are assertive usually mean that they are aggressive
   Strongly agree Agree Don't know Disagree Strongly disagree

50. I am very assertive
   Strongly agree Agree Don't know Disagree Strongly disagree

51. I am too assertive
   Strongly agree Agree Don't know Disagree Strongly disagree

52. I'm not sure that assertiveness is very important for health professionals
   Strongly agree Agree Don't know Disagree Strongly disagree

CHAPTER 12: SELF-AWARENESS SKILLS

53. Self-awareness is essential for health professionals
   Strongly agree Agree Don't know Disagree Strongly disagree

54. No-one is really very self-aware
   Strongly agree Agree Don't know Disagree Strongly disagree

55. I think that nobody can become truly self-aware
   Strongly agree Agree Don't know Disagree Strongly disagree

56. I would prefer it if I knew myself better
   Strongly agree Agree Don't know Disagree Strongly disagree

57. Other people know me better than I know myself
   Strongly agree Agree Don't know Disagree Strongly disagree

58. You can't teach people how to be self-aware
   Strongly agree Agree Don't know Disagree Strongly disagree

59. People I know tend to be more self-aware than me
   Strongly agree Agree Don't know Disagree Strongly disagree

60. Self-awareness is largely a question of learning from personal experience
   Strongly agree Agree Don't know Disagree Strongly disagree

There is no formal system for scoring this questionnaire although it is possible to devise one. One method would be to allocate a value to each of the statements thus:

32. I would prefer to handle my time more effectively

Strongly Agree	Agree	Don't Know	Disagree	Strongly Disagree
5	4	3	2	1

It should be noted that for some questions, the values should be reversed, thus:

22. I think counselling should be left to professionals

Strongly Agree	Agree	Don't Know	Disagree	Strongly Disagree
1	2	3	4	5

Once values had been allocated in this way, according to what are considered to be 'right' answers, the scores for each statement are added together and an overall score is obtained. This system may be of value if the questionnaire is used in a group setting or as a means of checking personal progress over a period of time. The real problem with this sort of scoring is establishing which answers are the 'right' ones. It is suggested that many of your responses to questions will depend on your own situation, your own values and your own preferences. For this reason, it is recommended that the questionnaire be used as a personal or small group instrument of reflection and not adapted for use as a research instrument without further validation.

Further reading

Adams, T. (1989) Dementia and family stress, *Nursing Times*, **85**, no. 38, 27-9.

Adams-Webber, J. and Mancusco, J.C. (eds) *Applications of Personal Construct Theory*, Academic Press, London.

Addison, C. (1980) Tolerating stress in social work practice: the example of a burns unit, *British Journal of Social Work*, **10**, 341-56.

Adler, R.B. (1977) *Confidence in Communication: A guide to assertive social skills*, Holt, Rinehart and Winston, London.

Adler, R. and Rodman, G. (1988) *Understanding Human Communication*, 3rd edn, Holt, Rinehart and Winston, New York.

Adler, R.B. and Towne, N. (1984) *Looking Out/Looking In: Interpersonal communication*, Holt, Rinehart and Winston, London.

Adler, R.B., Rosenfield, L.B. and Towne, N. (1983) *Interplay: The process of interpersonal communication*, Holt, Rinehart and Winston, London.

Alberti, R. (ed.) (1977) *Assertiveness: Innovations, applications, issues*, Impact, San Luis, Obispo, California.

Alberti, R.E. and Emmons, M.L. (1982) *Your Perfect Right: A guide to assertive living*, 4th edn, Impact Publishers, San Luis, California.

Allan, D.M.E., Grosswald, S.J. and Means, R.P. (1984) Facilitating self-directed learning, in J.S. Green, S.J. Grosswald, E. Suter and D.B. Walthall (eds) *Continuing Education for the Health Professions*, Jossey Bass, San Francisco, California.

Allan, J. (1989) *How to Develop Your Personal Management Skills*, Kogan Page, London.

Anderson, M., Chiriboga, D.A. and Bailey, J.T. (1988) Changes in management stressors on ICU nurses, *Dimensions of Critical Care Nursing*, **7**, no. 2, L 111-17.

Argyle, M (ed.) (1981) *Social Skills and Health*, Methuen, London.

Argyle, M. (1983) *The Psychology of Interpersonal Behaviour*, 4th edn, Penguin, Harmondsworth.

Argyris, C. (1982) *Reasoning, Learning and Action*, Jossey Bass, San Francisco.

Argyris, C. and Schon, D. (1974) *Theory in Practice: Increasing professional effectiveness*, Jossey Bass, San Francisco.

Arnold, E. and Boggs, K. (1989) *Interpersonal Relationships: Professional communication skills for nurses*, Saunders, Philadelphia.

Arnold, M.B. (1984) *Memory and the Brain*, Lawrence Erlbaum Associates, Hillsdale, New Jersey.

Ascott, M. (1988) Stress in the entertainment business, *Occupational Health*, **40**, no. 4, 520–23.

Ashworth, P. (1987) Technology and machines — Bad masters but good servants, *Intensive Care Nursing*, **3**, no. 1, 1–2.

Astbury, C. (1988) *Stress in Theatre Nurses*, Royal College of Nursing, London.

Atwood, A.H. (1979) The mentor in clinical practice, *Nursing Outlook*, **27**, 714–17.

Ausberger, D. (1979) *Anger and Assertiveness in Pastoral Care*, Fortress Press, Philadelphia.

Baddeley, D. (1983) *Your Memory: A User's Guide*, Penguin, Harmondsworth.

Baer, J. (1976) *How to Be Assertive (Not Aggressive): Women in life, in love and on the job*, Signet, New York.

Bailey, R. (1985) *Coping With Stress in Caring*, Blackwell, Oxford.

Bailey, R. and Clarke, M. (1989) *Stress and Coping in Nursing*, Chapman & Hall, London.

Baker, R. (1984) Stress in welfare work, *National Children's Home, Occasional Papers*, no. 5, 1–24.

Ball, M.J. and Hannah, K.J. (1984) *Using Computers in Nursing*, Reston Publishing, Reston, V.A.

Bannister, D. and Fransella, F. (1986) *Inquiring Man*, 3rd edn, Croom Helm, London.

Baruth, L.G. (1987) *An Introduction to the Counselling Profession*, Prentice Hall, Englewood Cliffs, New Jersey.

Bates, E. (1982) Doctors and their spouses speak: Stress in medical practice, *Sociology of Health and Illness*, **4**, no. 1, 25–39.

Belkin, G.S. (1984) *Introduction to Counselling*, Brown, Dubuque, Iowa.

Bellack, A.S. and Hersen, M. (eds) (1979) *Research and Practice in Social Skills Training*, Plenum Press, New York.

Benner, P. and Wrubel, J. (1989) *The Primacy of Caring: Stress and Coping in Health and Illness*, Addison Wesley, Menlo Park.

Bergman, A.B. (1988) Resident stress, *Paediatrics*, **82**, no. 2, 260–63.

Bernard, J.M. (1980) Assertiveness in children, *Psychological Reports*, **46**, 935–38.

Bibbings, J. (1987) The stress of working in intensive care: a look at the research, *Nursing*, **3**, no. 15, 567–70.

Bolger, A.W. (ed.) (1982) *Counselling in Britain: a reader*, Batsford Academic, London.

Bond, M. and Kilty, J. (1986) *Practical Methods of Dealing With Stress*, 2nd edn, Human Potential Research Project, University of Surrey, Guildford.

Boone, E.J., Shearon, R.W., White, E.E. *et al.* (1980) *Serving Personal and Community Needs Through Adult Education*, Jossey Bass, San Francisco, California.

Boud, D.J. (ed.) (1973) *Experiential Learning Techniques in Higher Education*, Human Potential Learning Project, University of Surrey, Guildford, Surrey.

Boud, D.J. and Prosser, M.T. (1980) Sharing responsibility: Staff-student cooperation in learning, *British Journal of Educational Technology*, **11**, no. 1, 24–35.

Boud, D.J., Keogh, R. and Walker, M. (1985) *Reflection: Turning Experience into Learning*, Kogan Page, London.

Boud, D.J. (ed.) (1981) *Developing Student Autonomy in Learning*, Kogan Page, London.

Bower, S.A. and Bower, G.H. (1976) *Asserting Yourself*, Addison Wesley, Reading, Mass.

Boydel, E.M. and Fales, A.W. (1983) Reflective learning: Key to learning from experience, *Journal of Humanistic Psychology*, **23**, no. 2, 99–117.

Bram, P.J. and Katz, L.F. (1989) A study of burnout in nurses working in hospice and hospital oncology settings, *Oncology Nursing Forum*, **16**, no. 4, 555–60.

Brandes, D. and Phillips, R. (1984) *The Gamester's Handbook*, Vol. 2, Hutchinson, London.

Brasweel, M. and Seay, T. (1984) *Approaches to Counselling and Psychotherapy*, Waverly, Prospect Heights.

Brookfield, S.D. (1986) *Understanding and Facilitating Adult Learning: A comprehensive analysis of principles and effective practices*, Open University Press, Milton Keynes.

Brookfield, S.D. (1987) *Developing Critical Thinkers: Challenging adults to explore alternative ways of thinking and acting*, Open University Press, Milton Keynes.

Broome, A. (1990) *Managing Change*, Macmillan, London.

Brown, A. (1979) *Groupwork*, Heinemann, London.

Brown, D. and Srebalus, D.J. (1988) *An Introduction to the Counselling Process*, Prentice Hall, Philadelphia, PA.

Brown, S.D. and Lent, R.W. (eds) (1984) *Handbook of Counselling Psychology*, Wiley, Chichester.

Brundage, D.H. and Mackeracher, D. (1980) *Adult Learning Principles and their Application to Program Planning*, Ministry of Education, Ontario.

Buber, M. (1958) *I and Thou*, Scribner, New York.

Buber, M. (1966) *The Knowledge of Man: a philosophy of the inter-human* (ed. M. Freidman), R.G. Smith (trans.), Harper and Row, New York.

Bugental, E.K. and Bugental, J.F.T. (1984) Dispiritedness: a new perspective on a familiar state, *Journal of Humanistic Psychology*, **24**, no. 1, 49–67.

Bugental, J.F.T. (1980) The far side of despair, *Journal of Humanistic Psychology*, **20**, 49–68.

Burnard, P. (1987) Spiritual distress and the nursing response: theoretical considerations and counselling skills, *Journal of Advanced Nursing*, **12**, 377–82.

Burnard, P. (1988) The heart of the counselling relationship, *Senior Nurse*, **8**, no. 12, 17–18.

Burnard, P. (1988) Stress and relaxation in health visiting, *Health Visitor*, **61**, no. 9, 272.

Burnard, P. (1988) Searching for meaning, *Nursing Times*, **84**, no. 37, 34–6.

Burnard, P. (1988) Preventing burnout, *Journal of District Nursing*, **7**, no. 5, 9–10.

Burnard, P. (1988) Coping with other people's emotions, *The Professional Nurse*, **4**, no. 1, 11–14.

Burnard, P. (1988) The spiritual needs of atheists and agnostics, *The Professional Nurse*, **4**, no. 3, 130–2.

Burnard, P. (1988) AIDS and sexuality, *Journal of District Nursing*, **7**, no. 2, 7–8.

Burnard, P. (1989) Counselling in surgical nursing, *Surgical Nurse*, **2**, no. 5, 12–14.

Burnard, P. (1989) The 'Sixth Sense', *Nursing Times*, **85**, no. 50, 52–3.

Burnard, P. (1989) *Teaching Interpersonal Skills: An experiential handbook for health Professionals*, Chapman and Hall, London.

Burnard, P. (1989) Exploring sexuality, *Journal of District Nursing*, **8**, no. 4, 9–11.

Burnard, P. (1989) Existentialism as a theoretical basis for counselling in psychiatric nursing, *Archives of psychiatric nursing*, **3**, no. 3, 142–7.

Burnard, P. (1989) Exploring nurses' attitudes to AIDS, *The Professional Nurse*, **5**, no. 2, 84–90.

Burnard, P. (1989) The nurse as non-conformist, *Nursing Standard*, **4**, no. 1, 32–5.

Burnard, P. (1990) Counselling the boss, *Nursing Times*, **86**, no. 1, 58–9.

Burnard, P. (1990) *Learning Human Skills: An experiential guide for nurses*, 2nd edn, Heinemann, Oxford.

Burnard, P. (1990) Counselling in crises, *Journal of District Nursing*, **8**, no. 7, 15–16.

Burnard, P. (1990) Recording counselling in nursing, *Senior Nurse*, **10**, no. 3, 26–7.

Burnard, P. (1990) Learning to care for the spirit, *Nursing Standard*, **4** no. 18, 38–9.

Burnard, P. and Morrison, P. (1989) Counselling attitudes in community psychiatric nurses, *Community Psychiatric Nursing Journal*, **9**, no. 5, 26–9.

Burnard, P. and Morrison, P. (1990) *Nursing Research in Action: Developing Basic Skills*, Macmillan, London.

Burton, A. (1977) The mentoring dynamic in the therapeutic transformation, *The American Journal of Psychoanalysis*, **37**, 115–22.

Callner, D. and Ross, S. (1978) The assessment and training of assertiveness skills with drug addicts: A preliminary study, *International Journal of the Addictions,* **13**, no. 2, 227–30.

Calnan, J. (1983) *Talking With Patients*, Heinemann, London.

Campbell, A. (1984) *Moderated Love*, S.P.C.K., London.

Campbell, A. (1984) *Paid to Care?* S.P.C.K., London.

Campbell, A.V. (1981) *Rediscovering Pastoral Care*, Darton, Longman and Todd, London.

Carkuff, R.R. (1969) *Helping and Human Relations*: Vol. I *Selection and Training*, Holt, Rinehart and Winston, New York.

Carlisle, J. and Leary, M. (1982) Negotiating groups, in Payne, R. and Cooper, C. (eds) *Groups at Work*, Wiley, Chichester.

Carson, B.V. (1989) *Spiritual Dimensions of Nursing Practice*, W.B. Saunders, Philadelphia.

Charles, J. (1983) When carers crash, *Social Work Today*, **15**, no. 12, 18–20.

Cheesebrow, D.J. (1987) Grid analysis for stress management, *Dimensions of Critical Care Nursing*, **6**, no. 5, 314–20.

Chene, A. (1983) The concept of autonomy in adult education: A philosophical discussion: *Adult Education Quarterly*, **32**, no. 1, 38–47.

Chenevert, M. (1978) *Special Techniques in Assertiveness Training for Women in the Health Professions*, C.V. Mosby, St Louis,

Chrousos, G.P., Loriaux, D.L. and Gold, P.W. (1988) *Mechanisms of Physical and Emotional Stress*, Plenum Press, New York.

Cianni-Surridge, M. and Horan, J. (1983) On the wisdom of assertive job-seeking behaviour: *Journal of Counselling Psychology*, **30**, 209–14.

Clark, C. (1978) *Assertive Skills for Nurses*, Contemporary Publishing, Wakefield, Mass.

Clark, M. (1978) Meeting the needs of the adult learner: Using non-formal education for social action, *Convergence*, **XI**, 3–4.

Claxton, G. (1984) *Live and Learn: An introduction to the psychology of growth and change in everyday life*, Harper and Row, London.

Clutterbuck, D. (1985) *Everybody Needs a Mentor: How To Further Talent Within an Organisation*, The Institute of Personnel Management: London.

Collins, G.C. and Scott, P. (1979) Everyone who makes it has a mentor,

Harvard Business Review, **56**, 89–101.

Cooper, C.L. (1981) *Stress Research*, Wiley, Chichester.

Cooper, C.L. and Marshall, J. (1980) *White Collar and Professional Stress*, Wiley, Chichester.

Cooper, C.L. and Payne, R. (eds) (1978) *Stress at Work*, Wiley, Chichester.

Cooper, C.L. and Payne, R. (1980) *Current Concerns in Occupational Stress*, Wiley, Chichester.

Corey, F. (1983) *I Never Knew I Had A Choice*, 2nd edn, Brooks-Cole, California.

Cormier, L.S. (1987) *The Professional Counsellor: a process guide to helping*, Prentice Hall, Englewood Cliffs, New Jersey.

Corsini, R. (1984) *Current Psychotherapies*, 3rd edn, Peacock, Itasca, Illinois.

Cunningham, P.M. (1983) Helping students extract meaning from experience, in R.M. Smith (ed.) *Helping Adults Learn How to Learn*, New Directions for Continuing Education No. 19, Jossey Bass, San Francisco.

Curtis, L., Sturm, G., Billing, D.R. and Anderson, J.D. (1989) At the breaking point: When should an overworked nurse bail out?, *Journal of Christian Nursing*, **6**, no. 1, 4–9.

Daleo, R.E. (1986) Taking care of the caregivers: Five strategies for stamina, *American Journal of Hospice Care*, **3**, no. 5, 33–8.

Daniels, V. and Horowitz, L.J. (1984) *Being and Caring: A psychology for living*, 2nd edn, Mayfield, Mountain View, California.

Darling, L.A.W. (1984) What do nurses want in a mentor?, *The Journal of Nursing Administration*, October, 42–4.

Davis, C.M. (1981) Affective education for the health professions, *Physical Therapy*, **61**, no. 11, 1587–93.

Dawley, H. and Wenrich, W. (1976) *Achieving Assertive Behaviour: A guide to assertive training*, Brooks/Cole, Monterey, California.

De Bono, E. (1982) *de Bono's Thinking Course*, BBC, London.

De Vito, J.A. (1986) *The Interpersonal Communication Book*, 4th edn, Harper and Row, New York.

Deckard, G.J. (1989) Impact of role stress on physical therapists' emotional and physical well-being, *Physical Therapist*, **69**, no. 9, 713–18.

de Leeuw, M. and de Leeuw, E. (1965) *Read Better Read Faster*, Penguin, Harmondsworth.

Dewe, P.J. (1989) Stressor frequency, tension, tiredness and coping: Some measurement issues and a comparison across nursing groups, *Journal of Advanced Nursing*, **14**, no. 4, 308–20.

Dickson, A. (1985) *A Woman in Your Own Right: Assertiveness and you*, Quartet Books, London.

Dilts, P.V. Jr. and Dilts, S.L. (1987) Stress in residency: Proposals for solution, *American Journal of Obstetrics and Gynaecology*, **157**, no. 5, 1093–6.

Distance Learning Centre (1986) *Stress in Nursing: an open learning study pack*, Distance Learning Centre, South Bank Polytechnic, London.

Dixon, D.N. and Glover, J.A. (1984) *Counselling: a problem solving approach*, Wiley, Chichester

Dobson, C.B. (1982) *Stress: The hidden anxiety*, MTP Press, Lancaster.

Dolan, N. (1987) The relationship between burnout and job satisfaction in nurses, *Journal of Advanced Nursing*, **12**, no. 1, 3–12.

Doswell, W.M. (1989) Physiological responses to stress, *Annual Review of Nursing Research*, **7**, 51–69.

Douglas, T. (1976) *Groupwork Practice*, Tavistock, London.

Dowd, C. (1983) Learning through experience, *Nursing Times*, 27th July, 50–2.

Downe, S. (1989) Prophets without honour — the burn — out of mid-wifery visionaries, *Midwives Chronicle*, **102**, no. 1214, 93–4.

Dryden, W., Charles-Edwards, D. and Woolfe, R. (1989) *Handbook of Counselling in Britain*, Routledge, London.

Duncan, S. and Fiske, D.W. (1977) *Face-to-Face Interaction: Research, methods and theory*, Lawrence Erlbaum Associates, Hillsdale, New Jersey.

Dusek, E.D. (1989) *Weight Management the Fitness Way: Exercise, Nutrition, Stress Control and Emotional Readiness*, Jones and Bartlett, London.

Edelwich, J. and Brondsky, A. (1980) *Burnout: Stages of disillusionment in the helping professions*, Human Sciences Press, New York.

Eden, D. (1982) Critical job events, acute stress and strain, *Organisational Behaviour and Human Performance*, **30**, 312–29.

Edmunds, M. (1983) The nurse preceptor role, *Nurse Practitioner*, **8**, no. 6, 52–3.

Egan, G. (1986) *Exercises in Helping Skills*, 3rd edn, Brooks/Cole, Monterey, California.

Ellis, A. (1962) *Reason and Emotion in Psychotherapy*, Lyle, Stuart, New Jersey.

Ellis, R. (ed.) (1989) *Professional Competence and Quality Assurance in the Caring Professions*, Chapman and Hall, London.

Ellis, R. and Whittington, D. (1981) *A Guide to Social Skill Training*, Croom Helm, London.

Epting, F. (1984) *Personal Construct Counselling and Psychotherapy*, Wiley, Chichester.

Ernst, S. and Goodison, L. (1981) *In our Own Hands: a book of self help therapy*, The Womens' Press, London.

Evans, D. (ed.) (1990) *Why Should We Care?*, Macmillan, London.

Everly, G.S. and Rosenfeld, R. (1981) *The Nature and Treatment of the Stress Response: a practical guide for clinicians*, Plenum Press, New York.

Fabry, J. (1968) *The Pursuit of Meaning*, Beacon Press, Boston, Mass.

Fagan, M.M. and Walter, G. (1982) Mentoring among teachers, *Journal of Educational Research*, **76**, no. 2, 113–18.

Farber, B.A. (ed.) (1983) *Stress and Burnout in the Human Services*, Pergamon Press, London.

Fay, A. (1978) *Making Things Better By Making Them Worse*, Hawthorne, New York.

Feldenkrais, M. (1972) *Awareness Through Movement*, Harper and Row, New York.

Fernando, S. (1990) *Mental Health, Race and Culture*, Macmillan, London.

Ferruci, P. (1982) *What We May Be*, Turnstone Press, Wellingborough.

Fielding, P. and Berman, P. (eds) (1989) *Surviving in General Management*, Macmillan, London.

Filley, A.C. (1975) *Interpersonal Conflict Resolution*, Scott, Foresman, Glenview, Illinois.

Fineman, S. (1985) *Social Work Stress and Intervention*, Gower, London.

Firth, J.A. (1985) Personal meanings of occupational stress: Cases from the clinic, *Journal of Occupational Psychology*, **58**, 139–48.

Firth, J.A. (1986) Levels and sources of stress in medical students, *British Medical Journal*, **292**, 1177–80.

Firth, H., McKeown, P., McIntee, J. and Britton, P. (1987) Burn-out, personality and support in long-stay nursing, *Nursing Times*, **83**, no. 32, 55–7.

Fisher, R. and Ury, W. (1983) *Getting to Yes: Negotiating Agreement without giving in*, Hutchinson, London.

Fisher, S. (1986) *Stress and Strategy*, Lawrence Erlbaum Associates, London.

Fisher, S. and Reason, J. (1988) *Handbook of Life Stress: Cognition and health*, Wiley, Chichester.

Foggo-Pays, E. (1983) *An Introductory Guide to Counselling*, Ravenswood, Beckenham.

Fontana, D. (1989) *Managing Stress*, British Psychological Society and Routledge, London.

Fordham, F. (1966) *An Introduction to Jung's Psychology*, Penguin, Harmondsworth.

Francis, D. and Young, D. (1979) *Improving Work Groups: A practical manual for team building*, University Associates, San Diego, California.

Frankl, V.E. (1959) *Man's Search for Meaning*, Beacon Press, New York.

Frankl, V.E. (1960) Paradoxical intention: a logotherapeutic technique, *American Journal of Psychotherapy*, **14**, 520–35.

Frankl, V.E. (1969) *The Will to Meaning*, World Publishing Co., New York.

Frankl, V.E. (1975) Paradoxical intention and dereflection: A logotherapuetic technique, *Psychotherapy: Theory, Research and Practice*, **12**, no. 3, 226–37.

Frankl, V.E. (1975) *The Unconscious God*, Simon and Schuster, New York.

Frankl, V.E. (1978) *The Unheard Cry for Meaning*, Simon and Schuster, New York.

Freeman, R. (1982) *Mastering Study Skills*, Macmillan, London.

French, P. (1983) *Social Skills for Nursing Practice*, Croom Helm, London.

Freudenberger, H. and Richelson, G. (1974) *Burnout: How to Beat the high cost of success*, Bantam Books, New York.

Fromm, E. (1941) *Escape from Freedom*, Avon, New York.

Geller, L. (1985) Another look at self-actualisation, *Journal of Humanistic Psychology*, **24**, no. 2, 93–106.

Gendlin, E. T. and Beebe, J. (1968) An experiential approach to group therapy, *Journal of Research and Developments in Education*, **1** 19–29.

George, P. and Kummerow, J. (1981) Mentoring for career women, *Training*, **18**, no. 2, 44–9.

Gibbs, G. (1981) *Teaching Students to Learn*, Open University, Milton Keynes.

Gibson, R.L. and Mitchell, M.H. (1986) *Introduction to Counselling and Guidance*, Collier Macmillan, London.

Gier, M.D., Levick, M.D. and Blazina, P.J. (1988) Stress reduction with heart transplant patients and their families: a multidisciplinary approach, *Journal of Heart Transplantation*, **7**, no. 5, 342–7.

Gilleard, C.J. (1987) Influence of emotional distress among supporters on the outcome of psychogeriatric day care, *British Journal of Psychiatry*, **150**, 219–23.

Glennerster, H. and Owens, P. (1990) *Nursing in Conflict*, Macmillan, London.

Goffman, I. (1971) *The Presentation of Self in Everyday Life*, Penguin, Harmondsworth.

Goldberg, L. and Beznitz, S. (1982) *Handbook of Stress: Theoretical and clinical aspects*, Macmillan, New York.

Gordon, S. and Waldo, M. (1984) The effects of assertive training on couples' relationships, *American Journal of Family Therapy*, **12**, 73–7.

Gormally, J. (1982) Evaluation of assertiveness: Effects of gender, rater involvement and level of assertiveness, *Behaviour Therapy*, **13**, 219–25.

Graham, N.M. (1988) Psychological stress as a public health problem: How much do we know?, *Community Health Studies*, **12**, no. 2, 151–60.

Haggerty, L.A. (1987) An analysis of senior nursing students' immediate responses to distressed patients, *Journal of Advanced Nursing*, **12**, no. 4, 451–61.

Halmos, P. (1965) *The Faith of the Counsellors*, Constable, London.

Hamilton, M.S. (1981) Mentorhood: a key to nursing leadership, *Nursing Leadership*, **4**, no. 1, 4–13.

Hanks, L, Belliston, L. and Edwards, D. (1977) *Design Yourself*, Kaufman, Los Altos, California.

Hanson, P. (1986) *The Joy of Stress*, Pan, London.

Hargie, O. (ed.) (1987) *A Handbook of Communication Skills*, Croom Helm, London.

Hargie, O., Saunders, C. and Dickson, D. (1981) *Social Skills in Interpersonal Communication*, 2nd edn, Croom Helm, London.

Harris, T. (1969) *I'm O.K., Your O.K.*, Harper and Row, London.

Hawkins, P. and Shohet, R. (1989) *Supervision and the Helping Professions*, Open University Press, Milton Keynes.

Health Education Authority: High Stress Occupation Working Party (1988) *Stress in the Public Sector: Nurses, police, social workers and teachers*, Health Education Authority.

Heginbotham, C. (1990) *Mental Health, Human Rights and Legislation*, Macmillan, London.

Heins, M., Fahey, S.N. and Leiden, L.I. (1984) Perceived stress in medical, law and graduate students, *Journal of Medical Education*, **59**, 169–79.

Hemmons, J. (1986) Stress in OH Nursing?, *Occupational Health*, **38**, no. 10, 328–30.

Herinck, R. (ed.) (1980) *The Psychotherapy Handbook*, New American Library, New York.

Heron, J. (1973) *Experiential Training Techniques*, Human Potential Research Project, University of Surrey, Guildford.

Heron, J. (1977) *Behaviour Analysis in Education and Training*, Human Potential Research Project, University of Surrey, Guildford, Surrey.

Heron, J. (1977) *Catharsis in Human Development*, Human Potential Research Project: University of Surrey, Guildford, Surrey.

Heron, J. (1978) *Co-Counselling Teachers Manual*, Human Potential Research Project, University of Surrey, Guildford.

Heron, J. (1980) *Paradigm Papers*, Human Potential Research Project, University of Surrey, Guildford.

Heywood-Jones, I. (1989) *Helping Hands*, Macmillan, London.

Heywood-Jones, I. (1990) *The Nurse's Code: A practical approach to the code of professional conduct*, Macmillan, London.

Hill, S.S. and Howlett, H.A. (1988) *Success in Practical Nursing in Personal Vocational Issues*, W.B. Saunders, Philadelphia, PA.

Hingley, P. and Cooper, C.L. (1986) *Stress and the Nurse Manager*, Wiley, Chichester.

Holt, R. (1982) An alternative to mentorship, *Adult Education*, **55**, no. 2, 152–6.

Houle, C.O. (1984) *Patterns of Learning*, Jossey Bass, San Francisco.

Howard, G.S., Nance, D.W. and Meyers, P. (1987) *Adaptive Counselling and Therapy: a systematic approach to selecting effective treatments*, Jossey Bass, San Francisco, California.

Howard, K. and Sharp, J.A. (1983) *The Management of a Student Research Project*, Gower, Aldershot.

Hughes, J. (1987) *Cancer and Emotion*, Wiley, Chichester.

Hull, D. and Schroeder, H. (1979) Some interpersonal effects of assertion, non-assertion and aggression, *Behaviour Therapy*, **10**, 20–9.

Hurding, R.F. (1985) *Roots and Shoots: a guide to counselling and psychotherapy*, Hodder and Stoughton, London.

Hutchins, D.E. (1987) *Helping Relationships and Strategies*, Brooks-Cole, Monterey, California.

Ivey, A.E. (1987) *Counselling and Psychotherapy: Skills, theories and practice*, Prentice Hall International, London.

Jacobson, D. (1989) Context and the sociological study of stress: an invited response to pearlin, *Journal of Health and Social Behaviour*, **30**, no. 3, 257–60.

James, M. and Jongeward, D. (1971) *Born to Win: Transactional analysis with gestalt experiments*, Addison-Wesley, Reading, Mass.

Jenkins, E. (1987) *Facilitating Self-Awareness: a learning package combining group work with computer assisted learning*, Open Software Library, Wigan.

Jenkins, J.F. and Ostchega, Y. (1986) Evaluation of burnout in oncology nurses, *Cancer Nursing*, **9**, no. 3, 108–16.

Johnson, D.W. (1972) *Reaching Out*, Prentice Hall, Englewood Cliffs, New Jersey.

Johnson, D.W. and Johnson, F.P. (1982) *Joining Together*, 2nd edn, Prentice Hall, Englewood Cliffs, New Jersey.

Jones, G. (1988) High-tech stress: Identification and prevention, *Occupational Health*, **40**, no. 9, 648–9.

Jones, J.G., Janman, K., Payne, R.L. and Rick, J.T. (1987) Some determinants of stress in psychiatric nurses, *International Journal of Nursing Studies*, **24**, no. 2, 129–44.

Jourard, S. (1964) *The Transparent Self*, Van Nostrand, Princeton, New Jersey.

Jourard, S. (1971) *Self-Disclosure: an experimental analysis of the Transparent Self*, Wiley, New York.

Jung, C.G. (1976) *Modern Man in Search of a Soul*, Routledge and Kegan Paul, London.

Kampel, W. and Kampel, M. (1988) Dental stress. The way it was/The way it is, *Alpha-Omega*, **81**, no. 1, 18–19.

Kavanagh, K.H. (1989) Nurses' networks: Obstacles and challenge, *Archives of Psychiatric Nursing*, **3**, no. 4, 226–33.

Keller, K.L. and Koening, W.J. (1989) Sources of stress and satisfaction in emergency practice, *Journal of Emergency Medicine*, **7**, no. 3, 293–9.

Kelly, C. (1979) *Assertion Training: A facilitator's guide*, University

205

Associates La Jolla, California.

Kennedy, E. (1979) *On Becoming a Counsellor*, Gill and Macmillan, London.

Kilty, J. (1978) *Self and Peer Assessment*, Human Potential Research Project, Guildford, UK.

Kilty, J. (1987) *Staff Development for Nurse Education: Practitioners Supporting Students: A report of a 5-day development workshop*, Human Potential Research Project, University of Surrey, Guildford.

King, E.C. (1984) *Affective Education in Nursing: A guide to teaching and assessment*, Aspen, Maryland.

Kizer, W.M. (1987) *The Health Workplace: A blueprint for corporate action*, Delmar, London.

Knowles, M.S. (1978) *The Adult Learner: A neglected species*, 2nd edn, Gulf, Texas.

Knowles, M. (1980) *The Modern Practice of Adult Education: From Pedagogy to Andragogy*, 2nd edn, Follett, Chicago.

Knowles, M.S. and Associates (1984) *Andragogy in Action: Applying Modern Principles of Adult Learning*, Jossey Bass, San Francisco, California.

Knox, A.B. (ed.) (1980) *Teaching Adults Effectively*, Jossey Bass, San Francisco, California.

Koberg, D. and Bagnal, J. (1981) *The Revised All New Universal Traveller: A soft-systems guide to creativity, problem-solving and the process of reaching goals*, Kaufmann, Los Altos, California.

Kopp, S. (1974) *If you Meet the Buddha on the Road, Kill Him!: A Modern Pilgrimage Through Myth, Legend and Psychotherapy*, Sheldon Press, London.

Kottler, J.A. and Brown, R.W. (1985) *Introduction to Therapeutic Counselling*, Brooks-Cole, Monterey, California.

L' Abate, L. and Milan, M. (eds) (1985) *Handbook of Social Skills Training and Research*, Wiley, New York.

Lachman, V.D. (1983) *Stress Management: a Manual for Nurses*, Grune and Stratton, Orlando, Florida.

Lang, A.J. and Jakubowski, P. (1978) *The Assertive Option*, Research Press, Champagne.

Larson, D.G. (1986) Developing effective hospice staff support groups: Pilot test of an innovative training program, *Hospice Journal*, **2**, no. 2, 41–55.

Lazarus, R.S. and Folkman, S. (1984) *Stress, Appraising and Coping*, Springer, New York.

Leady, N.K. (1989) A physiological analysis of stress and chronic illness, *Journal of Advanced Nursing*, **14**, no. 10, 868–76.

Leech, K. (1986) *Spirituality and Pastoral Care*, Sheldon Press, London.

Lennon, M.C. (1989) The structural contexts of stress: an invited response of pearlin, *Journal of Health and Social Behaviour*, **L 30**, no. 3, 261–8.

Lewis, H. and Streitfield, H. (1971) *Growth Games*, Bantam Books, New York.

Lewis, M. (1987) *Writing to Win*, McGraw Hill, London.

Liberman, R.P., King, L.W., DeRisi, W.J. and McCann, M. (1976) *Personal Effectiveness*, Research Press, Champagne.

Luft, J. (1984) *Group Processes: An Introduction to Group Dynamics*, 2nd edn, Mayfield, San Francisco.

Madders, J. (1980) *Stress and Relaxation*, Martin Dunitz, London.

Magrath, A., Reid, N. and Boore, J. (1989) Occupation stress in nursing, *International Journal of Nursing Studies*, **26**, no. 4, 343–58.

Marcer, D. (1986) *Biofeedback and Related Therapies in Clinical Practice*, Chapman and Hall, London.

Marshall, E.K. and Kurtz, P.D. (eds) (1982) *Interpersonal Helping Skills: A guide to training methods, programs and resources*, Jossey Bass, San Francisco, California.

Marson, S. (ed.) (1990) *Managing People*, Macmillan, London.

Matthews, D.A, Classen, D.C., Willms, J.L. and Cotton, J.P. (1988) A program to help interns cope with stresses in an internal medicine residency, *Journal of Medical Education*, **63**, no. 7, 539–47.

McCue, J.D. (1986) Doctors and stress: Is there really a problem? *Hospital Practice*, March, **30**, 7–16.

McGuire, J. and Priestley, P. (1981) *Life After School: A social skills curriculum*, Pergamon, Oxford.

McIntee, J. and Firth, H. (1984) How to Beat the Burnout, *Health and Social Services Journal*, 9th Feb., 166–8.

Meichenbaum, D. (1979) *Cognitive Behaviour Modification: an integrative approach*, Plenum Press, New York.

Meichenbaum, D. (1983) *Coping With Stress*, Century Publishing, London.

Meichenbaum, D. and Jaremko, M.E. (1983) *Stress Reduction and Prevention*, Plenum Press, New York.

Merriam, S. (1984) Mentors and proteges: a critical review of the literature, *Adult Education Quarterly*, **33**, no. 3, 161–73.

Meyeroff, M. (1972) *On Caring*, Harper and Row, New York.

Mezeiro, J. (1981) A critical theory of adult learning and education, *Adult Education*, **32**, no. 1, 3–24.

Michelson, L., Sugari, D., Wood, R. and Kazadin, A. (1983) *Social Skills Assessment and Training with Children*, Plenum Press, New York.

Middleton, J.F. (1989) Modifying the behaviour of doctors and their receptionists in recurrent stressful activity, *Journal of the Royal College of General Practitioners*, **39**, no. 319, 62–4.

Milne, D., Burdett, C. and Beckett, J. (1986) Assessing and reducing the stress and strain of psychiatric, *Nursing Times*, **82**, no. 19, 59–62.

Moore, D. (1977) *Assertive Behaviour Training: An annotated Bibliography*, Impact, San Luis Obispo, California.

Moreno, J.L. (1959) *Psychodrama Vol. II*, Beacon House Press, Beacon, New York.

Moreno, J.L. (1969) *Psychodrama Vol. III*, Beacon House Press, Beacon, New York.

Moreno, J.L. (1977) *Psychodrama, Vol. I*, 4th edn, Beacon House Press, Beacon, New York.

Morley, I.E. (1982) Preparation for negotiating: conflict, commitment and choice, in Bradstatter, H., Davis, J.H. and Stocker-Kreichgauer, G. (eds) *Group Decision Making*, Academic Press, London.

Morley, I.E. (1987) Negotiating and bargaining, in Hargie, O. (ed.) *A Handbook of Communication Skills*, Croom Helm, London.

Morsund, J. (1985) *The Process of Counselling and Therapy*, Prentice Hall, Englewood Cliffs, New Jersey.

Morton-Cooper, A. (1989) *Returning to Nursing: A guide for nurses and health visitors*, Macmillan, London.

Mouton, J.S. and Blake, R. R. (1984) *Synergogy: A new strategy for education, training and development*, Jossey Bass, San Francisco.

Muller, P.A. (1987) Avoiding burnout through prevention, *Journal of Post Anaesthetic Nursing*, **2**, no. 1, 53–8.

Munro, A., Manthei, B. and Small, J. (1988) *Counselling: The Skills of Problem-Solving*, Routledge, London.

Murgatroyd, S. (1986) *Counselling and Helping*, British Psychological Society and Methuen, London.

Murgatroyd, S. and Woolfe, R. (1982) *Coping with Crisis-Understanding and Helping Persons in Need*, Harper and Row, London.

Murphy, J.M., Nadelson, C.C. and Notman, M.T. (1984) Factors influencing first-year medical students perceptions of stress, *Journal of Human Stress*, **10**, 165–73.

Murphy, L.R. (1984) Occupational stress management: a review and appraisal, *Journal of Occupational Psychology*, **57**, 1–15.

Murphy, S.A. (1986) Perceptions of stress, coping and recovery one and three years after a natural disaster, *Issues in Mental Health Nursing*, **8**, no. 1, 63–77.

Myerscough, P.R. (1989) *Talking with Patients: A basic clinical skill*, Oxford Medical Publications, Oxford.

Nadler, L. (ed.) (1984) *The Handbook of Human Resource Development*, Wiley, New York.

Nash, E.S. (1989) Occupational stress and the oncology nurse, *Nursing*, **4**, no. 8, 37–8.

Nelson, M.J. (1989) *Managing Health Professionals*, Chapman and Hall, London.

Nelson-Jones, R. (1981) *The Theory and Practice of Counselling Psychology*, Holt Rinehart and Winston, London.

Nelson-Jones, R. (1984) *Personal Responsibility: counselling and therapy: an integrative approach*, Harper and Row, London.

Nelson-Jones, R. (1988) *Practical Counselling and Helping Skills: help-*

ing clients to help themselves, Cassell, London.

Nichols, K. and Jenkinson, J. (1990) *Leading a Support Group*, Chapman and Hall, London.

Nierenberg, G.I. (1973) *Fundamentals of Negotiation*, Hawthorn, New York.

Notman, M.T., Salt, P. and Nadelson, C.C. (1984) Stress and Adaptation in Medical Students: Who is most vulnerable?, *Comprehensive Psychiatry*, **25**, 355–66.

Nutall, P. (1982) Take me to your mentor, *Nursing Times*, **78**, no. 20, 826.

O'Dowd, T.C. (1987) To burn out or to rust out in general practice, *Journal of the Royal College of General Practice*, **37**, no. 300, 290–1.

Ohlsen, A.M., Horne, A.M. and Lawe, C.F. (1988) *Group Counselling*, Holt Rinehart and Winston, New York.

Onady, A.A., Rodenhauser, P. and Market, R.J. (1988) Effects of stress and social phobia on medical students' specialty choices, *Journal of Medical Education*, **63**, no. 3, 162–70.

Open University Coping With Crisis Group (1987) *Running Workshops: A guide for trainers in the helping professions*, Croom Helm, London.

Osborn, S.M. and Harris, G.G. (1975) *Assertive Training for Women*, Charles C. Thomas, Springfield, Illinois.

Palmer, M.E. and Deck, E.S. (1982) Assertiveness education: One method for teaching staff and patients, *Nurse Educator*, Winter, 36–9.

Payne, R. and Firth-Conzens, J. (eds) (1987) *Stress in Health Professionals*, Wiley, Chichester.

Pearlin, L.I. (1989) The sociological study of stress, *Journal of Health and Social Behaviour*, **L 30**, no. 3, 241–56.

Peplau, H.E. (1988) *Interpersonal Relationships in Nursing*, Macmillan, London.

Phelps, S. and Austin, N. (1975) *The Assertive Woman*, Impact, San Luis Obispo, California.

Phillip-Jones, L. (1982) *Mentors and Proteges*, Arbour House, New York.

Phillip-Jones, L. (1983) Establishing a formalised mentoring programme, *Training and Development Journal*, Feb, 38–42.

Pollack, K. (1988) On the Nature of Social Stress: production of a modern mythology, *Social Science and Medicine*, **26**, no. 3, 381–92.

Pope, B. (1986) *Social Skills Training for Psychiatric Nurses*, Harper and Row, London.

Porritt, L. (1990) *Interaction Strategies: An introduction for health professionals*, 2nd edn, Churchill Livingstone, Edinburgh.

Postman, N. and Weingartner, C.W. (1969) *Teaching as a Subversive Activity*, Penguin, Harmondsworth.

Priestley, P., McQuire, J., Flegg, D., Hemsley, V. and Welham, D. (1978) *Social Skills and Personal Problem Solving*, Tavistock, London.

Procter, B. (1978) *Counselling Shop: an introduction to the theories and techniques of ten approaches to counselling*, Deutsch, London.

Rankin-Box, D.F. (1987) *Complementary Health Therapies: A Guide for Nurses and the Caring Professions*, Chapman and Hall, London.

Rawlings, M.E. and Rawlings, L. (1983) Mentoring and networking for helping professionals, *Personnel and Guidance Journal*, **62**, no. 2, 116–18.

Reddy, M. (1987) *The Manager's Guide to Counselling at Work*, Methuen, London.

Roche, G.R. (1979) Much ado about mentors, *Harvard Business Review*, **56**, 14–28.

Rogers, C.R. (1951) *Client-Centred Therapy*, Constable, London.

Rogers, C.R. (1967) *On Becoming a Person*, Constable, London.

Rogers, C.R. (1983) *Freedom to Learn for the Eighties*, Merrill, Columbus.

Rogers, C.R. (1985) Toward a more human science of the person, *Journal of Humanistic Psychology*, **25**, no. 4, 7–24.

Rogers, C.R. and Stevens, B. (1967) *Person to Person: The problem of being human*, Real People Press, Lafayette, California.

Rogers, J.C. (1982) Sponsorship — Developing leaders for occupational therapy, *American Journal of Occupational Therapy*, **36**, 309–13.

Rogers, J.C. and Dodson, S.C. (1988) Burnout in occupational therapists, *American Journal of Occupational Therapy*, **42**, no. 12, 787–92.

Rowan, J. (1986) Holistic Listening, *Journal of Humanistic Psychology*, **26**, no. 1, 83–102.

Roy, I. (1973) *Structural Integration*, Viking Press, New York.

Russell, P. (1979) *The Brain Book*, Routledge and Kogan Paul, London.

Scammell, B. (1990) *Communication Skills*, Macmillan, London.

Schafer, B.P. and Morgan, M.K. (1980) An experiential learning laboratory: A new dimension in teaching mental health skills, *Issues in Mental Health Nursing*, **2**, no. 3, 47–57.

Scharer, K. (1988) Care for the care-giver, *Journal of the Association of Paediatric Oncology Nurses*, **5**, nos 1–2, 24.

Schmidt, J.A. and Wolfe, J.S. (1980) The mentor partnership: discovery of professionalism, *NASPA Journal*, **17**, 45–51.

Schon, D.A. (1983) *The Reflective Practitioner: How Professionals Think in Action*, Basic Books, Now York.

Schorr, T.M. (1978) The Lost Art of Mentoring, *American Journal of Nursing*, **78**, 1873.

Schulman, D. (1982) *Intervention in Human Services: A guide to skills and knowledge*, 3rd edn, C.V. Mosby, St Louis, Missouri.

Scott, W.P. (1986) *The Skills of Communicating*, Gower, Aldershot.

Shafer, P. (1978) *Humanistic Psychology*, Prentice Hall, Englewood Cliffs, New Jersey.

Shamian, J. and Inhaber, R. (1985) The concept and practice of preceptorship in contemporary nursing: A review of pertinent literature,

International Journal of Nursing Studies, **22**, no. 2, 79–88.

Shapiro, E.C., Haseltime, F, and Rowe, M. (1978) Moving up: Role models, mentors and the patron system, *Sloan Management Review*, **19**, 51–8.

Shaw, M.E. (1981) *Group Dynamics: The psychology of small group behaviour*, McGraw Hill, New York.

Shostak, A.B. (1980) *Blue-Collar Stress*, Addison-Wesley, Reading, Mass.

Shropshire, C.O. (1981) Group experiential learning in adult education, *Journal of Continuing Education in Nursing*, **12**, no. 6, 5–9.

Simon, S.B., Howe, L.W. and Kirschenbaum, H. (1978) *Values Clarification*, Revised edn, A. and W. Visual Library, New York.

Skevington, S. (ed.) (1984) *Understanding Nurses: The social psychology of nursing*, Wiley, Chichester.

Smith, E. and Wilks, N. (1988) *Meditation*, Macdonald and Co., London.

Smith, S. and Smith, C. (1990) *Personal Health Choices*, Jones and Bartlett, London.

Smith, T. (1984) Stress in the Prison Service, *Prison Service Journal*, October, 10–11.

Speizer, J.J. (1981) Role models, mentors and sponsors: The elusive concept, *Signs*, **6**, 692–712.

Stanfield, P. (1990) *Introduction to Health Professions*, 2nd edn, Jones and Bartlett, London.

Stevens, J.O. (1971) *Awareness: Exploring, Experimenting, Experiencing*, Real People Press, Moab, Utah.

Strauss, A. (1978) *Negotiations: Varieties, Contexts and Social Order*, Jossey Bass, San Francisco, California.

Sudman, S. and Bradburn, N.M. (1982) *Asking Questions: a practical guide to questionnaire design*, Jossey Bass, San Francisco, California.

Sweeney, M.A. (1985) *The Nurses Guide to Computers*, Macmillan, New York.

Tanner, D. (1986) *That's Not What I Meant!: How conversational style makes or breaks your relations with others*, Dent, London.

Taubman, B. (1976) *How to Become an Assertive Woman*, Simon and Schuster, New York.

Taylor, E. (1988) Anger intervention, *American Journal of Occupational Therapy*, **42**, no. 3, 147–55.

Taylor, S. (1986) Mentors: Who are they and what are they doing?, *Thrust For Educational Leadership*, **15**, no. 7, 39–41.

The Professional Nurse Developments Series (1990) *The Ward Sister's Survival Guide*, Austen Cornish, London.

The Professional Nurse Developments Series (1990) *Practice Check!*, Austen Cornish, London.

The Professional Nurse Developments Series (1990) *Effective Communication*, Austen Cornish, London.

The Professional Nurse Developments Series (1990) *Patient Education Plus*, Austen Cornish, London.

The Professional Nurse Developments Series (1990) *The Staff Nurse's Survival Guide*, Austen Cornish, London.

Thompson, J. (1989) Stress sense, *Nursing Times*, **85**, no. 21, 20.

Thygerson, A. (1989) *Fitness and Health: Lifestyle strategies*, Jones and Bartlett, London.

Torrington, D. (1982) *Face-to-Face in Management*, Prentice Hall, Englewood Cliffs, New Jersey.

Totton, N. and Edmonston, E. (1988) *Reichian Growth Work: Melting the blocks to life and love*, Prism Press, Bridport.

Tough, A.M. (1982) *Intentional Changes: A fresh approach to helping people change*, Cambridge Books, New York.

Trower, P. (ed.) (1984) *Radical Approaches to Social Skills Training*, Croom Helm, London.

Trower, P., O'Mahony, J.M. and Dryden, W. (1982) Cognitive aspects of social failure: Some implications for social skills training, *British Journal of Guidance and Counselling*, **10**, 176–84.

Truax, C.B. and Carkuff, R.R. (1967) *Towards Effective Counselling and Psychotherapy*, Aldine, Chicago.

Tschudin, V. (1986) *Counselling Skills for Nurses*, Baillière Tindall, London.

Tschudin, V. and Schober, J. (1990) *Managing Yourself*, Macmillan, London.

Vredenburgh, D.J. and Trinkaus, R.J. (1983) An analysis of role stress among hospital nurses, *Journal of Vocational Behaviour*, **22**, 82–95.

Wallace, W.A. (1986) *Theories of Counselling and Psychotherapy: a basic issues approach*, Allyn and Bacon, Boston.

Wallis, R. (1984) *Elementary Forms of the New Religious Life*, Routledge and Kegan Paul, London.

Watkins, J. (1978) *The Therapeutic Self*, Human Science Press, New York.

Weatley, D. (1981) *Stress and the Heart: Interactions of the Cardiovascular System*, Behaviour States and Psychotropic Drugs, Raven Press, New York.

Wheeler, D.D. and Janis, I.L. (1980) *A Practical Guide for Making Decisions*, Free Press, New York.

Whitaker, D.S. (1985) *Using Groups to Help People*, Tavistock/Routledge, London.

Wilkinson, J, and Canter, S. (1982) *Social Skills Training Manual: Assessment, programme design and management of Training*, Wiley, Chichester.

Winn, M.F. (1988) Imagery and the School Nurse, *Journal of School Health*, **58**, no. 3, 112–14.

Wlodkowski, R.J. (1985) *Enhancing Adult Motivation to Learn*, Jossey Bass, San Francisco, California.

Woodward, J. (1988) *Understanding Ourselves: The Uses of Therapy*, Macmillan, London.

Zajonc, R. (1980) Feelings and thinking: Preferences need no interference, *American Psychologist*, **35**, 151–75.

Zander, A. (1982) *Making Groups Effective*, Jossey Bass, San Francisco.

Zastrow, C. (1984) Understanding and Preventing Burnout, *British Journal of Social Work*, **14**, 141–55.

Index